100 Case Histories in Obstetri

counselling:
CUS /crur

- *prows*
- *gen th*
- *kidney cosremes.*

100 Case Histories in Obstetrics and Gynaecology

Michael D. G. Gillmer MA MD FRCOG
Consultant in Obstetrics and Gynaecology
John Radcliffe Hospital
Oxford
Honorary Lecturer
Nuffield Departments of Obstetrics and Gynaecology
University of Oxford

Philip J. Steer BSc MD FRCOG
Professor of Obstetrics and Gynaecology
Charing Cross and Westminster Medical School
West London Hospital
London

Julian Woolfson MB ChB FRCOG
Consultant in Obstetrics and Gynaecology
Queen Mary's Hospital
Sidcup
Kent

Churchill Livingstone

EDINBURGH LONDON MELBOURNE
NEW YORK AND TOKYO 1991

CHURCHILL LIVINGSTONE
Medical Division of Longman Group UK Limited

Distributed in the United States of America by
Churchill Livingstone Inc., 650 Avenue of the Americas,
New York, 10011, and by associated companies, branches
and representatives throughout the world.

First published 1991
   Reprinted 1992
   Reprinted 1994 (twice)

ISBN   0-443-02465-0

British Library Cataloguing in Publication Data
A catalogue record for this title is available
from the British Library

Library of Congress Cataloging in Publication Data
Gillmer, Michael.
   100 case histories in obstetrics and gynaecology/Michael D.G.
Gillmer, Philip Steer, Julian Woolfson.
      p.   cm.
   Includes index.

   1. Gynecology--Case studies.   2. Obstetrics--Case studies.
3. Gynecology--Examinations, questions, etc.   4. Obstetrics--
Examinations, questions, etc.   I. Steer, Philip.   II. Woolfson,
Julian.   III. Title.   IV. Title: One hundred case histories in
obstetrics and gynaecology.
   [DNLM: 1. Gynecology--case studies.   2. Gynecology--examination
questions.   3. Obstetrics--case studies.   4. Obstetrics--examination
questions.   WQ 18 G482z]
RG106.G54 1991
618.1'0076--dc20
DNLM/DLC
for Library of Congress   90-2508
                                                              CIP

                                                      The
                                                  publisher's
                                                 policy is to use
                                              **paper manufactured
                                              from sustainable forests**

Produced by Longman Singapore Publishers (Pte) Ltd
Printed in Singapore

Preface

Case histories form the basis of clinical medicine and those presented in this book reflect the accumulated obstetric and gynaecological experience of the authors, which exceeds 50 years.

The cases cover virtually all common obstetric and gynaecological disorders and also include a number of clinical curiosities. It is unlikely that any student whether undergraduate or postgraduate will see the full range of clinical problems that are presented in this book while in training. We therefore believe that it will serve to complement both clinical experience and the information contained in traditional textbooks.

Each case has been selected to entertain and educate the reader and to stimulate thought about diagnosis and management. The book provides ideal reading for all undergraduate and postgraduate students, especially those preparing for clinical and oral examinations, such as the DRCOG and MRCOG. It should also prove to be of interest to doctors in general practice.

We have enjoyed selecting these cases, which we believe highlight both the art and science of modern obstetric and gynaecological practice. We hope that you will enjoy reading them!

M.D.G.G.
P.J.S.
J.W.

Contents

Introduction

1 Taking and presenting a case history

Taking and presenting a good case history is both a science and an art. The science consists of asking the right questions in the right way to elicit the information you need from the patient in order to make the correct diagnosis. The art consists of presenting this data to others in a way which is both informative and interesting.

2 Asking the right question

There are certain basic questions which should be asked right at the beginning. Check the patient's name. This avoids much embarrassment if it turns out that you are reading the wrong GP referral letter. Ask her if she is married or single. Addressing women by the wrong title (Mrs, Miss or Ms) can easily cause offence. It also makes a significant difference to the interpretation of the history. For example, a single woman who has never had intercourse need not be asked about when she had her last smear.

Ask about her reproductive history. A good question to ask as a 'starter' is, 'Have you ever been pregnant?'. Forget the gravida para system. There is no agreement as to how these terms should be used, e.g. in relation to twin deliveries or stillbirths, and they can cause unnecessary confusion when the history is presented. Instead, ask about 'children, miscarriages and terminations' (the word abortion tends to mean miscarriage to doctors and termination to the lay public, and so is best avoided).

Always ask for the date of the last menstrual period. It is surprising how many otherwise good histories, even at postgraduate level, are marred by the omission of this vital information. I alway put it in the top right hand corner of the first page of my notes; an empty space there prompts me to ask it, and I always know where to find it later (very useful when writing up investigation forms, for example).

When you go on to the presenting complaint, do remember to define symptoms as best you can, e.g. with pain, ask about the site (asking the patient to point is a good way to define this, especially if their English is poor). Ask about severity (does it interrupt their work or sleep, make them double up, perspire or vomit?). Ask about precipitating, exacerbating and relieving factors.

When taking the supplementary history, e.g. about the urinary system, the questions will need to be focused depending on the presenting complaint. However, you should always ask about the following in gynaecology: vaginal discharge, intermenstrual bleeding, postcoital bleeding, and dyspareunia (in that order, it makes a logical way of introducing questions about the patient's sexual activity. Such questions should never be omitted, they often have direct diagnostic relevance, particularly in cases of possible pelvic infection, and even in prepubertal girls the question of sexual abuse cannot be igored). Contraception and the date of the last cervical smear should be asked about in women who are sexually active.

1

Always remember that in an examination situation you can continue asking about the history while you are performing parts of the examination, e.g. putting on the blood pressure cuff or testing the urine. Once you have learnt to do this it can also be very helpful in a busy clinic!

3   Presenting the right data

This is where the art comes in. Do not simply present the history as a verbatim account of the way you took it. This could be done by a tape recorder. It is your job as a doctor to interpret the data and present it in a processed and digested way so that the listener can assimilate the facts easily. Try and imagine that your listener (an audience, or an examiner) is hearing a radio play. Paint a picture in words which is interesting, is in a logical sequence and which is easy on the ear. The best way to present data is in time order, as this is the way most people live their lives! It is hard on an audience to tell them all about a pregnancy, and then throw in the fact that the woman has mitral stenosis right at the end! They have to go back and readjust their interpretation of the history in the light of this vital information, which is not easy to do.

It is therefore best to give a brief summary of the case to start with, so that the listener has some idea what it is all about, and then build up the picture in a logical, time-ordered sequence. If it is essential to the understanding of why someone has presented with abdominal pain to know that she has already had three laparoscopies demonstrating the presence of endometriosis, then start with the first presentation and laparoscopy, not with the most recent presenting complaint.

Don't clutter up your history with irrelevant routine findings. However, do include 'positive negatives'. For example, it is not necessary to say 'the JVP [jugular venous pressure] was not raised' in a history relating to acute pyelonephritis, but it is an important point if the patient has a pregnancy complicated by mitral stenosis.

Explain the significance of the history and examination findings as you go along. Say, 'because she has mitral stenosis I checked the rhythm of the pulse, but it was regular and there was no evidence of atrial fibrillation'. This demonstrates your knowledge to the examiner and educates the less sophisticated audience.

Try to make your presentation easy to listen to and therefore to assimilate. Don't read your notes rapidly in a monotone in an attempt to get the whole thing over as fast as possible. By all means use notes, but vary your tone of voice, and look up regularly to see if the audience is keeping up with you. Speak at the audience, not at a screen or at the wall, and don't speak through your hand. Try not to say 'um' too often. This requires a little practice—which is the only way to make yourself perfect!

Finally, end with a summary and, if you can, a conclusion as to the differential diagnosis. If you can suggest a prognosis and possible therapy, so much the better, but only do this if you are fairly sure about them. If not, allow these points to emerge in the discussion which should follow a good presentation.

4 How to find references

The first reference source to which 'the novice' is usually directed when he begins to research a particular topic is the *Index Medicus*. He is then taken aback by the complexity of this source and the number of references available, not to mention the frequent difficulty of finding some of the journals indexed! Experience, however, shows that there are simpler and more practicable ways to review the literature. Such a system is outlined below.

(a) References in obscure journals are often very difficult to find. Furthermore, once obtained, it is often difficult for the novice to judge their scientific value. It is usually better to start with well known and authoritative journals. These have the following advantages:

(i) Competition for publication in the major journals is considerable. This makes it likely that only papers with a significant contribution to make appear in them.

(ii) Papers are carefully refereed for scientific merit and validity, and the editor will ensure that they are comprehensible.

(iii) The journals are likely to be readily available even in quite small postgraduate libraries.

The four major obstetrical and gynaecological journals are:

The British Journal of Obstetrics and Gynaecology
The American Journal of Obstetrics and Gynaecology
Obstetrics and Gynaecology (USA)
Obstetrical and Gynaecological Survey (USA)

In addition, most UK graduates will subscribe to the *British Medical Journal*, and hopefully read it fairly thoroughly each week. This serves to keep one up to date with general developments in medicine, but, in addition, a number of important articles on obstetrics and gynaecology appear from time to time. It is a good idea to keep some sort of index of these articles so that they may be retrieved readily at a later date.

(b) Make sure you are clear in your own mind as to the scope of the subject you wish to research. Then scan each of the five journals mentioned above for a paper on this subject or a closely related topic. Most papers start with a brief review of their subject and end with a list of references. These references will have been carefully selected by the authors as being relevant to the subject under discussion and will form a useful initial reading list. In this way, one paper will lead to another, also with a list of references, and quickly a reference list of 40–50 titles will build up.

It is unlikely that a topic of significant importance will not be represented in one of the five journals within the last year or so. But bear in mind that if your subject is very specialised, e.g. a particular type of rare ovarian cancer, you should scan any article on malignant ovarian disease in general, rather than expecting to find an article devoted entirely to this subject.

This technique will also ensure that you do not miss any important recent articles. This often occurs when using a reference index, which is inevitably a few months out of date. It will usually provide sufficient information for a case discussion, or brief review.

(c) If you need more information, or you do not find enough in the journals listed above, a number of additional sources should be scrutinised.

    (i) *The British Journal of Hospital Medicine*: this frequently has articles on important aspects of obstetrics and gynaecology. Some topics (e.g. management of labour) recur regularly every four years or so. These review articles are a rich source of references to more detailed work. The last four or five years of this monthly journal should therefore be scrutinised for an issue with a suitable review article.

    (ii) Textbooks held by your local library: undergraduate texts, or even postgraduate texts covering a wide range, are not usually a very rich source of references. Specialised texts on more specific subjects, e.g. the cervix, may well contain more detailed information and appropriate references (although these will inevitably be a few years out of date).

(d) Try and think of a colleague or superior who takes a special interest in the subject or related topics. They will often be able to suggest useful references, and may even have a prepared reference list.

(e) Write to, or phone the secretary of, a well known research worker in the field. If you ask courteously, and *explain your reason for wanting the information*, most workers will oblige with half a dozen references or more, or may send a copy of their latest review article on the subject.

(f) If you have any difficulty in finding the journal or book you need, or wish general advice, always ask your local librarian. Most welcome the opportunity to help with specific data collection tasks; it makes a break from their routine and enables them to practice the skills in which they have been trained. They will also be able to help you in the use of the specialised reference sources.

(g) *Index Medicus*, and related sources, e.g. the *Bibliography of Reproduction*, and *Bibliography of Medical Reviews*, are usually issued monthly, and are compiled using computer techniques. You will already have seen most of the readily accessible articles if you have followed the scheme outlined above. Articles on 'extraspecialised' topics can be obtained by your librarian from the British National Library. This will involve photocopying and postal charges, which are usually nominal. If you are using these sources for the first time you should always enlist the aid of the librarian.

(h) Computer searches. Cross checks on a wide range of subjects can be made using the 'key-words' system. The commonest available system is 'Medline'. Access will have to be arranged by your librarian. It is used 'on-line' for material indexed in the last two years or 'off-line' for material indexed since 1966. Searches can be carried out at:

Science Reference Library
(Bayswater Branch)
10, Porchester Gardens
Queensway
London W2 4DE
Tel. no: 071-727 3022 ext. 65

or
Central Information Services
University of London Library
Senate House
Malet Street
London, WC1E 7HE
Tel. no: 071-636 4515 ext. 937

   Searches may be requested by telephone, by letter, or in person
(it is necessary to make an appointment first). Both libraries make
a charge, which is (at the time of writing) approximately £5 for the
search and 1 pence extra for each reference found. If you make
your topic too broad, you will obtain a vast number of references,
which will be both expensive and confusing. Your librarian will
help you to frame your request properly. Do not expect such
searches to be totally comprehensive. Experienced research
workers who use these systems regularly estimate that about 50%
of the worthwhile references in any subject can be tracked down
using computer search techniques, the rest will have to be found
by detective work as described in sections 1 - 5 above.

Obstetrics 1

A Kenyan Asian factory worker had come to England when she was 17 years old. Three years later a marriage was arranged with a carpenter who came from India to join her. When she was 23 years old she became pregnant for the first time and she was seen in the antenatal clinic after 15 weeks of amenorrhoea. She spoke little English, but with the help of an interpreter it was established that she had always had a regular 28-day cycle since her menarche and there was no history of any medical disorder. In particular, she had not suffered from tuberculosis.

On examination she was 156 cm tall and weighed 43.5 kg, giving her a body mass index (weight in kilograms divided by height in metres squared) of 17.9. Her blood pressure was 100/50 and routine urinalysis was normal. Her uterus was thought to be consistent with only 9 weeks gestation. Haemoglobin concentration was 12.8 g/dl with an MCV of 86 fl.

A routine fetal anomaly scan was carried out at 17 weeks of amenorrhoea and showed a biparietal diameter (BPD) of 32.5 mm and a head circumference (HC) of 12.1 cm (equivalent to the mean for 15 weeks). A further scan 2 weeks later was consistent with the first and, in addition, showed an abdominal circumference (AC) of 12.2 cm.

She was subsequently seen monthly and at first her progress was normal. At 29 weeks of amenorrhoea she weighed 49 kg. Her blood pressure was 100/55 and Hb 13.2 g/dl (MCV 85fl). Her further progress was as follows (Table 1):

Table 1

Weeks of amenorrhoea	Gestation by initial scan	Fundal height (cm)	Weight (kg)	BPD (mm)	HC (cm)	FAC (cm)
29	27	24	49			
31	29	25	49	76	24.5	22.0
33	31	26	48			
35	33	27	49			
36	34	27	48.5	82.5	28.0	25.5
37	35	28	49			
38	36	29	49	84.0	28.2	26.1
39	37	29	49			

Two standard deviations below the mean for BPD at 36 weeks is 90 mm, for HC 30 cm and for AC 28 cm. The presentation was cephalic throughout. Vaginal examination at 39 weeks of amenorrhoea revealed the cervix to be 2 cm dilated, anterior, and soft with a canal length of 1 cm and the station of the presenting part 2 cm above the spines (Bishop score 7).

1. What conclusions can you draw from this information?
2. What further investigations are indicated?
3. Outline your preferred management.

1. This woman's fetus is clearly at high risk of intrauterine growth retardation (IUGR). Not only is she of low body weight (<45 kg), but she is also underweight for her height (the normal body mass index is from 19 to 24). A low body mass index approximately doubles the risk of IUGR. She also has a low blood pressure, which is more common in underweight women who produce small babies. Her Hb concentration is high for a pregnant Asian woman (Asians are often vegetarian, and tend therefore to have low iron stores). This suggests a less than optimal plasma volume expansion (plasma volume expansion in pregnancy is known to correlate well with fetal growth).

   Between 18 and 34 weeks of gestation, fundal height in centimetres corresponds well to the weeks of gestation if the fetus is growing normally (±3 cm should be allowed to take account of variations in maternal anatomy). If the fundal height in centimetres is 4 or more less than the weeks of amenorrhoea, then there is a 60% chance of IUGR. In this case, the fundal height was already 3 cm less than the ultrasound gestation at 27 weeks, indicating the need for close monitoring. When, at 31 weeks by ultrasound, the fundal height was 5 cm behind, monitoring by regular scan estimation of fetal size was commenced. The persistent finding of values more than two standard deviations below the mean for gestational age is associated with an 8-fold increase in the likelihood of IUGR.

   Failure of weight gain is also an important warning sign for IUGR in women of normal or below normal body weight. This contrasts to the situation in overweight women (body mass index >30, weight >80 kg), where weight gain shows little or no correlation with birth weight. Weight gain should be assessed in terms of the pattern over the whole pregnancy. Small fluctuations in weight from week to week are common, particularly towards term when the rate of weight gain slows, mirroring the pattern of fetal growth. Thus if overall weight gain is normal, a small drop in weight from one week to the next is not significant unless it becomes progressive over two to three weeks.

   The pattern of the ultrasound measurements in this fetus suggests a chronic, symmetrical form of IUGR. There are many causes of this type of IUGR, ranging from fetal anomaly (such as trisomy) through fetal infection with viruses such as rubella and cytomegalovirus (CMV) to nutritional deprivation. This latter diagnosis is the most likely in the present case, associated with the reduced maternal body mass index and her failure to gain weight. A similar pattern may be seen in maternal organic disease, such as severe hypertension or systemic lupus erythematosus (SLE), but there was no evidence of such an aetiology in the present case.

2. Further ultrasound diagnostic tests which can be applied in IUGR include the biophysical profile and Doppler waveform velocimetry of the umbilical and uterine circulations. The biophysical profile includes, besides the above measurements of BPD, HC and AC, estimates of liquor volume (usually measured as the depth of the largest fluid pocket), fetal breathing activity, movement and tone, and the pattern of the antenatal cardiotocogram. Doppler velocimetry is no better than the above measurements in

assessing likely centile birthweight, but absent end-diastolic velocities do indicate an increased likelihood of significant fetal and neonatal complications, including polycythaemia and necrotising enterocolitis.

3. The decision to deliver a baby with IUGR is inevitably a compromise, depending on the gestation. The more mature the baby, the less is the indication necessary to prompt delivery. Such indications include failure of the fetus to show growth on ultrasound over two consecutive weeks, and repetitive abnormalities of the fetal heart rate pattern. In any case, in the presence of established IUGR, it is probably wise not to allow the pregnancy to go past term, when placental function may deteriorate. In addition, a favourable cervix, indicating the probability of a successful induction of labour with the chance of vaginal birth, tilts the balance in favour of delivery, particularly after 36 weeks gestation. The fetus must be monitored as carefully as possible in labour, as it is at increased risk of intrapartum asphyxia. Even if the indication for delivery is an abnormal fetal heart rate pattern, induction of labour should be considered, as 60% of such fetuses show adaptation during labour with a return to normal of the heart rate pattern.

In this case, a further scan at 38 weeks by ultrasound dates showed no further growth and labour was therefore induced by artificial rupture of the membranes (ARM) and intravenous oxytocin infusion monitored by measurement of intrauterine pressure. The CTG was normal throughout the first stage of labour, but there was a sudden and persistent bradycardia in the second stage. Delivery was therefore expedited with Simpson's forceps. The male infant weighed only 2.18 kg, which is less than the third centile for 38 weeks. His Apgar scores were 7 at 1 minute and 10 at 5 minutes. The cord artery pH was 7.24 with a base deficit of 9 mmol/l. The infant subsequently progressed well.

Obstetrics 2

A 29-year-old social worker, Mrs R P, was married to a policeman. Born in the United States of America, she was 14 years old when her soldier father was posted to England. She had remained in England following her marriage, although her family had returned to the USA. Her medical history included a laminectomy at the age of 17, and three attacks of cystitis following her marriage at the age of 23. Full investigation of these attacks (including intravenous urography) revealed no abnormality and subsequently she had no further infections. She had commenced a combined oral contraceptive 'pill' at the age of 22, and had discontinued this 4 months before she attended the booking clinic with 8 weeks amenorrhoea. A pregnancy test was positive.

Booking examination revealed a reddish granular area on the upper third of the anterior wall of the vagina. Scraping the area with an Ayre's spatula showed it to have a nodular, sandpaper-like consistency and produced a small amount of bleeding. The cervix itself was small and only about 0.5 cm long. It was, however, closed and firm. A cervical smear was taken.

The cervical smear report showed CIN 3; the smear from the vagina was normal.

Writing to Mrs R P's mother in the USA elicited that, because of a threatened abortion, she had taken oral diethyl stilboestrol when she was pregnant with Mrs R P. She had taken 5 mg daily from 9 weeks gestation, increasing by 5 mg a day every 2 weeks until by 17 weeks she was taking 25 mg a day. Thereafter she increased the dosage by 5 mg at weekly intervals so that at 35 weeks she was taking 115 mg per day. She then discontinued the medication.

1. Describe a likely cause for the attacks of cystitis.
2. What condition is responsible for the abnormality noted in the vagina?
3. How is it related to the cervical lesion?
4. What complications may occur during the pregnancy?
5. Discuss further management.

1. The attacks of urinary infection may well have been associated with the beginning of sexual activity. This phenomenon is often termed 'honeymoon cystitis' and is thought to be due to mild trauma to the urethra caused by the exuberant intercourse which is common in new sexual relationships.

2. Mrs R P has vaginal adenosis, which is caused by intrauterine exposure to diethyl stilboestrol (DES). Between 1948 and 1971, DES, a non-steroidal synthetic oestrogen was prescribed for an estimated 2.5 million pregnant women, most of them in the USA. Indications were threatened or habitual abortion, previous stillbirth or premature labour, pre-eclampsia, essential hypertension, and diabetes. The rationale for the use of DES was based on work by Smith and Smith (1949)[1], who postulated that stilboestrol stimulated the placenta to produce increased amounts of both oestrogen and progesterone. Use of DES stopped abruptly in 1971 when an association was noted between exposure to it in utero and later development of clear cell adenocarcinoma of the vagina. Fortunately, this risk is now estimated to be not higher than 1 in 700 exposed women, and it may be as low as 1 in 7000. Nonetheless, between a quarter and a half of DES exposed women have structural abnormalities of the cervix and vagina (such as transverse ridges, a cervical hood, endocervical pseudopolyps and cervical hypoplasia) and about two-thirds have uterine anomalies on hysterosalpingography.

3. In 1974 Stafl and Mattingly[2] hypothesised that because of the extensive transformation zone on the cervix and in the vagina of many DES exposed women, they might be at increased risk of developing squamous cell carcinoma. Current evidence suggests that this is not so, and the simultaneous presence of vaginal adenosis and CIN in this case is therefore simply coincidental.

4. Once pregnancy has occurred in DES exposed women, there are two main complications which can occur. Firstly, the incidence of ectopic pregnancy is increased to about 3%, possibly because of abnormalities in the structure of the fallopian tube. Secondly, if the pregnancy is intrauterine, there is a one in four chance of preterm delivery.

5. In the present case it was easy, using ultrasound, to demonstrate the presence of a live fetus in utero. The prophylaxis of preterm delivery was problematical, as it was felt that the cervix was too deficient for a MacDonald cervical suture to be effective. Mrs R P was not willing to accept the more extensive surgery involved in a Shirodkar suture, particularly since it was not possible to give a definite assurance that it would be effective. Two-weekly cervical assessment was therefore performed to monitor cervical competence. At 28 weeks gestation, the cervix had softened and admitted

[1]Smith O W & Smith G Van S 1949 New England Journal of Medicine 241:562

[2]Stafl A & Mattingley R F 1974 American Journal of Obstetrics and Gynaecology 120:666

a finger tip; Mrs R P was accordingly admitted to hospital for rest. At 31 weeks, the cervix had dilated to 3 cm. Dexamethasone, 12.5 mg, was given I/M and repeated 12 hours later. Three days later, she went into labour and after 3 hours produced a live female infant weighing 1.5 kg. The baby progressed well.

Two months postpartum the cervical CIN persisted and was removed to a depth of 5 mm using a carbon dioxide laser.

Obstetrics 3

A 23-year-old English housewife booked at 12 weeks of amenorrhoea in her first pregnancy. She was normotensive, 1.62 m tall and weighed 55 kg. A scan confirmed her gestation. By the time she was 14 days past her estimated date of delivery, she weighed 72 kg and was still normotensive. Abdominal palpation showed the fetus to be in cephalic presentation, with four-fifths of the fetal head palpable. Ultrasound scanning showed a normally situated placenta and no obvious fetal anomalies. The cervix was unripe, with a Bishop score of only 2. It was decided to induce labour, the indication being 'postmaturity'. An erect lateral pelvimetry showed normal dimensions (minimum diameter 11.8 cm). Because the cervix was unfavourable, prostaglandin E_2 pessaries were used in an attempt to ripen the cervix. Three pessaries (3 mg each) were used at 12-hour intervals, with no change in the cervix. An artificial rupture of the membranes was then performed, and intravenous oxytocin infusion was started. It was commenced at 2 mu/min and increased by 2 mu/min every 15 minutes up to a maximum rate of 12 mu/min. Over the first 4 hours, uterine activity was in the upper normal range (1274 ± 372 kPas/15 min), 164 Montevideo Units (MU) with a contraction frequency of 4 in 10 minutes and a mean active pressure of 41 mmHg. In the first 4 hours following the commencement of the oxytocin infusion the cervix dilated from 1 cm to 5 cm. However, over the next 8 hours, uterine activity declined to 950 + 310 kPas/15 min despite an increase in the oxytocin infusion rate to 32 mu/min, and the cervix only dilated to 7 cm. No further progress was made over the next 12 hours, and so, after a total labour of 24 hours, a lower segment caesarean section was performed. A live male infant was delivered weighing 3.5 kg, in excellent condition (Apgar scores 9, 10).

Three years later Mrs D presented again in her second pregnancy. She was confirmed by scan to be 18 weeks gestation. She was normotensive and weighed 67 kg. Her pregnancy progressed normally until at her estimated date of delivery she weighed 76 kg. The fetal head had been free throughout the pregnancy with the presentation varying from cephalic, five-fifths palpable, to oblique, with the head in the iliac fossa. The cervix remained unfavourable, with a Bishop score of 4.

1. Comment on the decision to induce labour in her first pregnancy.
2. What precautions are advisable when inducing labour with prostaglandin pessaries?
3. Was the pelvimetry of any value?
4. Outline your further management of the second pregnancy.

1. Induction of labour for 'postmaturity' (variably defined as more than 40, 41, or 42 weeks of pregnancy) was fashionable from the late 1960s to the late 1970s and is still practised in some units. The justification usually put forward is that 'unexpected mature stillbirths of unknown cause' are thereby avoided. As perinatal surveillance of the fetus and understanding of perinatal pathology has improved, this category of stillbirth has largely disappeared. While some cases of failing placental function are avoided by induction, there is (as in this case) always the risk of failed induction. The more modern approach is to view postmaturity as an indication for detailed antenatal monitoring of the fetus. A typical scheme would be to commence a fetal movements count ('kick chart') at 40 weeks, perform an ultrasound scan at 41 weeks to exclude as far as possible clinically undetected IUGR associated with oligohydramnios, and start daily cardiotocography at 42 weeks (this involves only a small proportion of the population).

2. When the cervix is unfavourable, vaginal prostaglandins are probably the agents of choice for the induction of labour: in most cases they ripen the cervix, thereby reducing the risk of failed induction in primigravidae from approximately 40% to about 15%. The main problem with induction of labour using prostaglandin pessaries is that the effects are somewhat unpredictable. In most cases, uterine contractions are produced, which may asphyxiate the compromised fetus, so that continuous fetal heart rate monitoring is advisable following administration of the pessaries. However, 40% of primigravidae fail to establish progressive labour even after two pessaries 6 –12 hours apart, so that monitoring may need to be very prolonged. In contrast, precipitate delivery may occur with few premonitory signs, so that expert paediatric care should be available at all times following administration. In rare cases, tumultuous uterine activity is produced, so that urgent caesarean section is necessary to safeguard the fetus. Facilities for emergency caesarean section should therefore always be on hand.

3. Since it is now usual practice to allow almost all mothers with a cephalic presentation a carefully monitored 'trial of labour', routine X-ray pelvimetry is unnecessary even if the head remains unengaged prior to the onset of labour.

4. In the second pregnancy the mother was allowed to go into spontaneous labour, which she did at 4 days after her due date. She progressed from 2 to 10 centimetres dilatation over 7 hours. Uterine activity was normal throughout (mean 1216 + 525 kPas/15 min). No oxytocin was required. Crossmatched blood was kept available. After a second stage of 2 hours, a Simpson's forceps delivery was performed of a female infant weighing 3.46 kg. Apgar scores 8, 10. The uterine scar was confirmed to be intact after delivery (although such an assessment is not necessary as a routine).

Obstetrics 4

A 25 year-old doctor's receptionist first became pregnant 6 months after her second marriage. Her husband was a despatch rider. She habitually smoked 35 cigarettes a day, but reduced this to 15 when she found she was pregnant.

She booked at 15 weeks of amenorrhoea, a gestation confirmed by clinical examination and ultrasound scanning. She was 1.64 metres tall and weighed 74 kg. By 1 week after her estimated date of delivery, she weighed 84 kg. She remained normotensive. She was admitted in spontaneous labour at 21.00 hours. The cervix was soft, thin, fully effaced, posterior and 2 centimetres dilated. The presentation of the fetus was cephalic, with the presenting part 1 centimetre above the spines.

By 10.15 hours the following day, the cervix was 5.5 cm dilated, but then by 15.15 hours no further dilatation had occurred. Uterine activity was poor (650 kPas/15 min) and so an oxytocin infusion was commenced to a maximum of 6 mu/min. An epidural anaesthetic was given at 17.00 hours.

By 22.50 hours, the cervix was fully dilated. The continuous fetal heart rate recorded by cardiotocograph showed a normal pattern (baseline rate 140 beats/minute, variability — 10 beats/minute, accelerations present with only small — less than 30 beats/minute — decelerations synchronous with contractions), but the liquor was noted to be meconium stained. Vaginal examination revealed a deflexed occipito-posterior (OP) presentation, with the lowest part of the fetal head 1 cm below the spines. There was little moulding, no head was palpable per abdomen, and clinically the pelvis felt roomy. Milne Murray forceps were applied but there was no descent with traction.

1. What is the significance of the meconium staining of the liquor?
2. What are the implications of the fact that the fetal head is engaged in the pelvis?
3. Why was the attempt at delivery with Milne Murray forceps unlikely to be successful?
4. How would you deliver the patient?

1. Meconium staining of the liquor is a common response of the mature fetus to the stress of labour. It is very uncommon if the fetus is less than 34 weeks gestation, but the incidence rises with advancing fetal maturity so that a third of normal fetuses in labour at 42 weeks gestation will pass meconium. At any gestation, the proportion of fetuses passing meconium will increase if they are subjected to abnormal stresses. Meconium staining in preterm labour is a particularly worrying sign, and may indicate intrauterine infection (such as with *Listeria monocytogenes*). In the 'post-dates' fetus, a variety of abnormal stresses can increase the proportion of fetuses passing meconium, including head compression, cord compression, acute hypoxia (e.g. associated with epidural-induced hypotension) and chronic hypoxia and acidosis. It is therefore an indication for careful monitoring, preferably by cardiotocography, and fetal blood sampling and pH estimation if the heart rate pattern is abnormal. In this case, the cardiotocograph tracing indicated that the passage of meconium was due to reflex stress rather than hypoxia.

2. The fact that the fetal head was engaged indicated that the malpresentation was not due to absolute disproportion at the pelvic inlet. This meant that, if the pelvic outlet was normal (which can be assessed with some accuracy by clinical examination, unlike the inlet), a vaginal delivery was feasible if the malpresentation could be corrected. This proposition was supported by the relative lack of moulding.

3. The attempt at delivery without rotation, using the Milne Murray forceps, was unlikely to be successful because the head was occiput posterior; the abnormal presentation was therefore due to deflexion of the head which will be made worse by direct traction (the occiput was impacted in the hollow of the sacrum, providing a pivotal point for extension of the head).

4. In view of the absence of asphyxia (shown by the normal cardiotocogram) and the engaged head with little moulding, it was felt that vaginal delivery would be possible if the head was rotated to occipito-anterior. This rotation was accompanied with ease, with the aid of a general anaesthetic (an epidural would be a good alternative) and Kielland's forceps. Moderate traction then flexed the head and a female infant weighing 3.16 kg and Apgar scores of 4 at 1 minute and 9 at 5 minutes was delivered (the low 1 minute Apgar was probably related to the general anaesthetic; there was no indication of acidosis). Elective intubation was performed to aspirate meconium from the trachea, the baby had an uneventful neonatal period with no suggestion of meconium aspiration.

Obstetrics 5

A 32-year-old Irish shop assistant was married to a carpenter. She booked in her first pregnancy at 12 weeks gestation, weighing 54.5 kg. She was 1.65 metres tall. By 40 weeks gestation she weighed 70.5 kg. She had remained normotensive throughout the pregnancy.

Her main anxiety during the pregnancy had been that her husband had been taking prednisone 5 mg daily and thalidomide, for a skin complaint, at the time of conception. To allay her fears, regular ultrasound scanning had shown normal fetal growth, with no obvious abnormalities of the skeletal system.

She was admitted in spontaneous labour 12 days after her estimated date of delivery. Initial vaginal examination at 07.00 hours revealed the cervix to be soft, mid-position, fully effaced, and 3.5 cm dilated. The presenting part was, however, still high (3 cm above the spines) and a fetal electrode was not placed. Fetal heart rate monitoring was commenced using an ultrasound transducer, with a normal trace being produced. At 10.00 hours, the cervix was still only 4 cm dilated and an intrauterine catheter was introduced to measure uterine activity, which was normal. The presenting part had descended to 2 cm above the spines, and a face presentation was diagnosed. At 15.00 hours, repeat examination revealed that the presentation had become a brow, left mento-anterior. Because a technically satisfactory trace was not being obtained via ultrasound, a fetal electrode was placed, as high up on the forehead as possible. By 17.00 hours the tracing showed a baseline tachycardia of 165 beats/minute (previously 130 beats/minute) with a baseline variability of only 3–4 beats/minute and some synchronous decelerations of 20 beats/minute amplitude. The cervix was fully dilated, the presenting part was 1 cm above the spines, and three-fifths of the head was palpable per abdomen.

1. What was the risk to the fetus of its father taking thalidomide at the time of conception?
2. Describe the investigation you would have liked to do to help you in the management of the labour described above, and give your opinion as to why it was not done.
3. List the causes of brow presentation.
4. What do you think was done next in the case described above?

1. Thalidomide was introduced in 1956 to West Germany, and in 1958 to Great Britain, marketed as a sedative. It causes phocomelia (reduction deformities of the arms and legs), as well as abnormalities of the eyes, ears, heart, alimentary and urinary tracts, when taken by the mother in the first trimester of pregnancy. There is no known effect on spermatogenesis and ingestion by the father does not cause these abnormalities in his offspring. The drug was withdrawn from the general market by the end of 1961, but is still available for specific indications such as the treatment of erythema nodosum leprosum.

2. Probably the most helpful investigation in the above situation would have been fetal blood sampling and pH estimation, to see if the abnormal trace represented fetal hypoxia leading to a significant acidosis. It was not done because the presentation precluded access to the fetal scalp. It might have been possible to obtain a sample from the forehead, but in view of the dangerous proximity of the eyes, and the risk of permanent scarring (particularly important if the baby was female), it was decided not to pursue this test. X-ray investigation is traditional in some centres, but it was not carried out in this case for a number of reasons. Firstly, it is difficult to obtain satisfactory quality X-rays in labour because of maternal restlessness. The abnormal presentation would in any case be sufficient to preclude vaginal delivery despite normal pelvic dimensions. Secondly, the detection of fetal abnormalities from X-rays taken in labour is notoriously unreliable, and in any case this fetus had been extensively scrutinised with ultrasound before the onset of labour. Finally, the use of X-rays carries a slight long-term maternal and fetal risk of leukaemia.

3. Face and brow presentations are associated with a higher rate of fetal abnormality than would be expected by chance. The direct cause of the abnormal presentation (leaving aside rare tumours of the thyroid) is usually said to be increased tone in the posterior muscles of the neck — why this should occur in connection with fetal anomaly is unknown. Other factors associated with brow presentation include a lax uterus and pendulous abdomen, a contracted pelvis, multiple pregnancy, dolichocephaly, and a dead fetus.

4. Because the fetal head remained unengaged, and the cardiotocography tracing suggested developing fetal compromise, it was decided to deliver by caesarean section. This was uneventful, and resulted in the delivery of a live female, weight 3.5 kg, with Apgar scores of 5 at 1 minute and 9 at 5 minutes. Mother and daughter progressed well in the puerperium.

Obstetrics 6

A South African Asian entered the United Kingdom at the age of 20. While working as a shop assistant, she married an Asian radio/TV engineer from India. Both were Hindu. Three years later she became pregnant for the first time. At booking, she was 1.52 m tall and weighed 48 kg. She had 14 weeks of amenorrhoea, and an early ultrasound confirmed her period of gestation. By 38 weeks she had gained 10 kg. She went into spontaneous labour at this gestation. In the first 9 hours of labour, the cervix dilated from 1.5 cm to 5 cm, but then failed to dilate further over the next 8 hours. Her uterine activity was normal, with a mean level of 1300 kPas/15 min (contractions of 8 kPa — 60 mmHg — every 4 minutes). A lower segment caesarean section was performed for secondary arrest of cervical dilatation. A female infant weighing 2.18 kg was delivered with Apgar scores of 4 and 9 at 1 and 5 minutes respectively.

The pelvimetry on the 10th postpartum day showed the following dimensions (Table 2) :

Table 2

			Lower limit of normal
Inlet	Conjugate	10.6 cm	(10.2)
	Available transverse	12.2 cm	(12.4)
Cavity	Lower AP	11.6 cm	(11.4)
	Interspinous	11.0 cm	(10.1)
Outlet	Posterior sagittal	8.9 cm	(10.1)
	Subpubic angle	96°	(81°)

In her next pregnancy 18 months later, she booked at 10 weeks of amenorrhoea. Gestation was confirmed by scan. Her weight was 47 kg and this increased to 60 kg at 38 weeks. Serial ultrasound cephalometry showed growth of the biparietal diameter and abdominal circumference along the 10th centile. At 38 weeks, presentation was cephalic, but the head remained high, with four-fifths palpable in the abdomen, as it had been throughout the previous month. The scans showed an upper segment placenta.

1. Discuss the relevance of her Hindu religion.
2. Was her first baby growth retarded?
3. How would you manage her from 38 weeks onwards in her second pregnancy?

1. The Hindu religion eschews the eating of animals. Although some believers will eat products which do not require the killing of the animal (milk and cheese, for example) the cow is especially sacred and therefore dairy products are often 'taboo'. Many strict Hindus are exclusively vegan. This may lead to dietary deficiency, particularly of iron (causing anaemia), vitamin D (leading to rickets) and protein (leading to a reduced lean body mass, and potentially to growth retardation of the fetus). All Hindus should therefore have a careful dietary history taken at booking, and should be assessed critically for signs of malnutrition. Iron and folic acid supplements should be given routinely, and vitamin D and protein supplements (conveniently available as soya bean products) given as necessary.

2. The diagnosis of growth retardation in the neonate should be, strictly speaking, a dynamic one based on metabolic factors such as the presence of hypoglycaemia and hypothermia, with assessment of energy reserves such as subcutaneous fat and liver glycogen. The categorisation of the neonate by birthweight alone is controversial for the following reasons:
   (i)   Differing standards are required for male and female infants (approximately 150 g difference in mean birthweight at term).
   (ii) It is now usual to correct for gestation age.
   (iii) The influence of maternal height and weight is considerable, with bigger mothers generally having bigger babies, and vice versa. However, the functional significance of this difference is uncertain; babies born to small mothers may be smaller solely due to genetic factors, or the overall incidence of retarded growth in this group may be increased.
   (iv) Different ethnic groups have different 'normal' distributions of birthweight, but there is disagreement as to whether this reflects genetic variation in growth potential, or differences in overall nutritional standards leading to a higher incidence of genuine growth retardation in some populations. Nonetheless, the first baby in this case was less than the 3rd centile, weight for gestational age, and thus had at least a 50% chance of showing intrapartum or neonatal dysfunction compatible with the diagnosis of 'growth retardation'.

3. In some countries, for example the USA, it is usual to recommend 'once a caesarean, always a caesarean'. However, in the UK, standard practice is to recommend a 'trial of scar' provided that it is known that the initial caesarean was lower segment. An X-ray pelvimetry is commonly recommended to exclude gross degrees of pelvic contracture. In the present case, the dimensions of the pelvis, although slightly reduced, were reasonable for the size of fetus expected. In addition, the pelvis widened towards the outlet, suggesting that once the fetus had negotiated the inlet further progress would be straightforward. The most important factors promoting a vaginal delivery in the second labour are efficient uterine activity and rapid cervical dilatation. This is most likely to occur in spontaneous labour. In addition, the dangers of uterine rupture from hyperstimulation if prostaglandins or oxytocin are used are completely avoided if labour is spontaneous. In the present case, spontaneous labour ensued 10 days before the due

date. At the onset of labour the cervix was 3 cm dilated. Steady progress was made over the next 16 hours, to full dilatation. Oxytocin was not used to accelerate the rate of progress because intrauterine pressure measurement showed uterine activity to be normal. A spontaneous delivery ensued, of a live male, weighing 2.62 kg (just below the 10th centile, weight for gestational age), with Apgar scores of 8 and 10 at 1 and 5 minutes.

Obstetrics 7

An 18-year-old unmarried West Indian woman first attended the antenatal clinic at 16 weeks gestation in her third pregnancy. She had had therapeutic terminations of pregnancy in her first two pregnancies, at 9 and 14 weeks of gestation respectively. There were no medical complications following the terminations, which were performed by suction evacuation following dilatation of the cervix under general anaesthesia.

She had left school at the age of 15, as had her 19-year-old consort. Neither had been gainfully employed since leaving school. She was currently smoking 15 cigarettes per day, and had recently finished a course of antibiotics prescribed by her family doctor for 'bronchitis', which she attributed to her damp accommodation. The family doctor had also treated her three times in the previous year for 'urinary tract infections'.

The 'booking' examination and investigations were unexceptional (she was sickle negative), apart from a pure growth of *Escherischia coli* resistant to penicillin and ampicillin. There were also 100 white cells per high power field on microscopy. She was treated with nitrofurantoin 100 mg four times daily.

At 19 weeks gestation, she reattended with a severe ulcerative vulvitis, and herpes virus was cultured from a swab taken from one of the ulcers. She was treated symptomatically with analgesics.

At 24 weeks gestation, she attended the labour ward as an emergency one weekend, complaining of lower abdominal pain and dysuria. She was apyrexial and on examination the uterus and abdomen were non-tender, and the fetal heart was heard.

1. What aspects of the history would you like clarified?
2. What further examination(s) would you perform, and why?
3. What investigations are appropriate?
4. Would you send her home on antibiotics?

1. When any pregnant woman presents with abdominal pain, the history noted must include the presence or absence of nausea/vomiting, shoulder pain, bowel function (constipation, diarrhoea, passage of mucus or blood per rectum) and the presence or absence of vaginal discharge (purulent, watery, irritant) or bleeding, (fresh — bright red, old — dark red, amount). In the present case there were no additional symptoms other than a 48-hour history of increasing watery discharge.

2. This woman has many factors in her history which put her at risk of preterm labour (young, single and unsupported, smoker, recurrent urinary tract infections, two previous terminations of pregnancy, and a sexually transmitted disease contracted in early pregnancy). Therefore, an assessment of whether this episode of abdominal pain represents preterm labour must be made — starting with an examination of the cervix. This should initially be done via a Cuscoe's speculum, when high vaginal and cervical swabs can be taken. Nitrazine ('amnistix') can be used to assess vaginal pH as an aid to deciding whether the amniotic membranes are ruptured. If the cervix is not obviously dilated, a gentle digital assessment should be made to determine its effacement, dilatation and consistency. A mid-stream specimen of urine should also be examined immediately for organisms and white cells, and sent for culture. An ultrasound examination is sometimes useful to detect conditions such as hydramnios. Cardiotocography can also be helpful in the evaluation of uterine activity.

3. The obvious potential mistake here is to assume this lady has another urinary tract infection. It is only too easy to ascribe lower abdominal pain in pregnancy, which is common, to urinary tract infection, which is also common. However, this should never be done without the supporting evidence of finding organisms and white cells in the urine, and preferably obtaining a positive culture. Even then, a positive finding does not exclude the possibility of premature labour, since urinary tract infections are associated statistically with an increased risk of preterm delivery.

4. The correct course is therefore to investigate this woman both for urinary tract infection *and* for preterm labour. She proved to have a cervix which was 5 cm dilated, with the amniotic membranes bulging through. She went on inevitably to abort. The baby weighed only 550 g and died shortly after delivery. There was no evidence of urinary tract infection on this occasion.

Obstetrics 8

A 20-year-old West Indian secretary booked at 15 weeks gestation in her first pregnancy. She was unmarried, but had a stable relationship with her labourer boyfriend. At booking she was 1.66 m tall and weighed 68 kg. Her pregnancy was uneventful, and at term she weighed 79 kg. The fetus was clinically judged to be of normal size and was in cephalic presentation. She went into spontaneous labour at 12 days past her EDD. The cervix was favourable at the onset of labour (Bishop score 9, dilatation 3 cm) and she progressed well so that 4 hours later the cervix was 8 cm dilated. At that time, it was noted that the liquor had become stained with thick, fresh meconium. Continuous fetal heart rate recording from a scalp electrode showed a baseline tachycardia of 165 beats/minute, with good baseline variability (8 beats/minute) and some accelerations. There were, however, variable decelerations with contractions, amplitude 60 beats/minute, lasting 40 seconds. A fetal blood sample showed a pH of 7.31 (mean of three estimates). One hour later the cervix was fully dilated, and the fetal head was occipito-anterior at the spines, with marked caput and ++ moulding (reducible overlapping of the skull bones). The fetal heart rate pattern was unchanged except for a reduction of baseline variability to only 4 beats/minute. A repeat fetal blood sample showed a pH of 7.29. The liquor continued to be meconium stained.

1. Discuss the possible aetiologies of the meconium staining of the liquor.
2. Discuss the risks to which this baby was exposed.
3. Outline your management of the second stage.

1. The passage of meconium by the fetus is usually a reflex event, and therefore depends upon the maturity of the innervation of the bowel. Passage of meconium is very unusual before 34 weeks gestation, and when it occurs in the preterm fetus, the possibility of infection (e.g. with *Listeria monocytogenes*) should be considered. On the other hand, almost a third of fetuses at 42 weeks gestation will pass meconium. There can be no doubt that stress can stimulate the passage of meconium, but this need not be an asphyxial stress; in many cases, meconium staining of the liquor will be associated with an apparently normal fetus with a normal neonatal outcome.

    In the present case, it seems likely that the fetus is passing meconium because (i) it is very mature and (ii) because of head compression activating the meconium reflex. The evidence for fetal head compression lies in the marked variable fetal heart rate decelerations and the ++ moulding. The fetal blood sample pH results suggested that there was no severe or chronic asphyxia, and indeed cord blood-gas values confirmed this : cord venous blood, pH 7.33, Po_2 19 mmHg (2.5 kPa), Pco_2 31 mmHg (4.1 kPa), bicarbonate 16.2 mmol/l, base excess - 6.3 mmol/l; cord arterial blood, pH 7.28, Po_2 12 mmHg (1.6 kPa), Pco_2 43 (5.7 kPa), bicarbonate 20 mmol/l, base excess - 3.3 mmol/l.

2. The main risk to which this baby was exposed was meconium aspiration. This was most likely to occur if (i) the pharynx was full of meconium stained liquor at the time of birth, (ii) there was an acute asphyxial stress causing gasping. There was also a possibility that the prolonged head compression was beginning to compromise cerebral blood flow, suggested by the reduction in baseline fetal heart rate variability. Other side effects of prolonged head compression include cephalhaematoma.

3. In view of the abnormal fetal heart rate and the meconium staining of the liquor, most obstetricians would consider elective forceps delivery to have a number of advantages. Firstly, the asphyxial potential of the second stage is minimised, and secondly the delivery can be carefully controlled. The paediatrician should be present to aspirate the pharynx as soon as the baby's head is born. There are of course iatrogenic risks (mostly trauma) from a forceps delivery, but in this case the favourable station and position means that delivery should be straightforward. Facilities for intubation and resuscitation must be available in case they are needed; intubation and aspiration via the endotracheal tube are advisable if inspection with the laryngoscope shows meconium below the cords despite careful aspiration of the pharynx before delivery of the baby's body. It would also be wise to have facilities for caesarean section readily available, since, in the remote event of the forceps delivery not being successful, the fetus will now be at major risk and should be delivered abdominally without delay.

Obstetrics 9

A 39-year-old Ghanaian woman booked at the antenatal clinic at 14 weeks gestation in her fourth pregnancy.

Her hospital records revealed that she first came to medical attention aged 23, when she was admitted with what seemed like acute pyelonephritis. However, investigation revealed that she was having a 'sickling crisis'. Haemoglobin electrophoresis showed the pattern of HbSC, rather than the more common HbSS.

Her first pregnancy, aged 25 was also complicated by a sickling crisis, at 37 weeks gestation. She was treated with sodium bicarbonate orally (5 mg tds), folic acid (5 mg tds), and intravenous Rheomacrodex and heparin. She was given pethidine for pain. She was also given a 2-pint blood transfusion. She delivered a healthy male infant weighing 3.5 kg at 39 weeks gestation.

In her second pregnancy, aged 28, she had a prolonged spontaneous labour, and needed augmentation with an oxytocin infusion. She delivered another healthy male weighing 3.5 kg. Her haemoglobin level dropped to 7.8 kg/dl in the puerperium, and she was transfused with 2 pints of blood.

Aged 32, she had an uneventful termination of pregnancy at 8 weeks gestation, for social reasons (her marriage was breaking up).

Aged 39, she booked at 17 weeks gestation, having acquired a new partner. He was also Negro, and an urgent haemoglobin electrophoresis showed him to have a sickle trait.

1. What is the chance of the child having sickle disease?
2. Describe how you would counsel the couple?
3. What is the current preferred management of sickle crisis?
4. From what other abnormality is the child at increased risk?

1. The child has a 50% chance of having sickle disease (25% SS, 25% SC) and a 50% chance of having either sickle trait (HbS) or HbC trait.

2. In the developed countries, the couple should be counselled that antenatal tests now exist to diagnose sickle disease in utero. The first test that was developed involved fetoscopy and fetal blood sampling (usually from a vessel at the insertion of the umbilical cord into the placenta) at 18–20 weeks gestation. Most fetal blood red cells contain HbF, but normally there is a small admixture (3.5–7.5%) of adult haemoglobins, HbA_1, and HbA_2. If only HbS is detected, the child has sickle disease (or, in this case, HbSC disease). Although this test cannot be done readily before 18 weeks gestation, the result can be obtained within a few hours of the fetal blood sampling being carried out. However, the risk of fetal loss due to the procedure is 2–5%.

   More recently, the technique of gene probe analysis using DNA restriction endonucleases has made it possible to detect the absence of the gene for HbA_1 synthesis in fetal cells cultured from an amniotic fluid sample. Amniocentesis can be done as early as 12–14 weeks; however, cell culture to provide sufficient material for gene probe analysis takes about two weeks. The fetal loss rate from amniocentesis is probably not more that 0.5%.

   Transcervical or transabdominal chorionic villus aspiration at 6–12 weeks gestation usually provides sufficient fetal material for culture and analysis, and is now available at most perinatal centres; fetal loss rates are probably about 1–2%.

   The test performed will therefore depend on the gestation at which the couple present for diagnosis. Should sickle disease be diagnosed, the couple would normally be offered termination of pregnancy. Before proceeding with the test, the risks of the procedures (particularly fetal loss rate) should be discussed, and the techniques with their associated discomforts explained in detail. The couple's attitude to therapeutic abortion should be explored since the tests are normally only carried out if they would accept termination if the child was found to have sickle disease. They should be informed fully as to the prognosis for sickle disease, and it should be explained that, although often a crippling disease, it can sometimes be relatively benign (in perhaps 20% of cases).

3. The modern management of sickle disease relies upon blood transfusion to dilute the abnormal cells with healthy ones. Good oxygenation is also vital. Bicarbonate and low molecular weight dextrans are not now thought to be of major importance. Prophylactic transfusion in pregnancy is favoured by some authorities.

4. The child has a 1 in 140 risk of having Down's syndrome, due to the mother's advanced age (population average 1 in 700). Chromosomal analysis to detect this syndrome should therefore also be offered.

Obstetrics 10

A 15-year-old schoolgirl was admitted via casualty to the labour ward. She was previously 'unbooked', but appeared to be about 36 weeks pregnant. She was accompanied by her Spanish boyfriend, who worked as a waiter. The couple revealed that they had been at a 'glue sniffing' session when the girl started to experience abdominal pain. There had been no vaginal bleeding or loss of liquor.

On examination, the uterus was non-tender, the fetal heart rate was normal, and the cervix was 5 cm dilated. Urgent investigations showed a haemoglobin concentration of 8.6 g/dl, blood group O Rh positive.

Labour progressed rapidly to full dilation 1 1/2 hours later. Artificial rupture of the membranes was then carried out, and at 03.52 hours a spontaneous vertex delivery of a live female weighing 2.4 kg occurred after a second stage of only 10 minutes. The third stage was managed actively and the placenta was removed complete. A small midline perineal tear had occurred, which was sutured with catgut.

Mother and baby were transferred to the postnatal ward, but at 05.50 hours the senior house officer was asked to see her because of continued vaginal bleeding. On examination, she was pale with a pulse rate of 120 beats/min, and a blood pressure of 110/60 mmHg. She was complaining of lower abdominal pain, but examination revealed a well contracted uterus which was only moderately tender. The rest of the abdomen was soft and bowel sounds were normal.

1. Discuss how you would manage this situation.
2. What are the common causes of primary postpartum haemorrhage?
3. What is meant by 'active management' of the third stage?

1. The postnatal ward is not a good place for the investigation of pastpartum haemorrhage, particularly at night. The beds are not conducive to thorough examination (particularly vaginal), the lighting is often poor and staffing levels are low. The patient was therefore returned to the labour ward for investigation. Prior to transfer, an intravenous infusion of normal saline was set up, and blood sent for crossmatching (4 units requested).

    Once in the labour ward, observations of pulse and blood pressure were continued, and a thorough examination was carried out in the lithotomy position. Speculum examination of the vagina allowed the evacuation of 500 ml of blood clots, with confirmed fresh bleeding from the upper vagina. Because of the lack of patient co-operation, largely due to inadequate analgesia, a general anaesthetic was administered. The whole genital tract was then examined thoroughly by inspection with a powerful light and by digital exploration. This showed that the vagina and uterus were intact, but the cervix felt ragged. Using three sponge-holding forceps, advancing them round the cervix one at a time, several large cervical lacerations were demonstrated with a bleeding vessel at the base of each one.

    A blood transfusion was commenced, and the bleeding vessels underrun with catgut sutures to obtain haemostasis. In view of the low haemoglobin on admission, and an estimated loss of at least 1 litre of blood, 4 units of blood were transfused over the next 12 hours.

2. The commonest cause of primary postpartum haemorrhage is uterine atony. This will usually respond to intravenous oxytocics. Lacerations of the genital tract (vaginal, paravaginal, cervix and uterine) are the next commonest, but often overlooked. A sinister cause is failure of normal coagulation, which can occur following placental abruption, fulminating pre-eclampsia, or septicaemia (inherited coagulopathies are very rare in women).

3. Active management of the third stage involves using an oxytocic (usually 5 units of oxytocin and 0.5 mg of ergometrine intramuscularly) to accelerate contraction and retraction of the uterus. To avoid trapping the placenta, controlled cord traction is necessary to remove the placenta as soon as it has separated from the uterus. (Separation is not achieved by pulling on the cord, but by contraction of the uterus. Failure to appreciate this point can result in snapping of the cord, haemorrhage, or uterine inversion.) This method has been shown in a large prospective randomised controlled trial to minimise blood loss from postpartum haemorrhage, and to reduce the need for blood transfusion by at least half compared with physiological management without oxytocics. Side effects of the oxytocics are rare, with nausea and vomiting being mainly due to the ergometrine. Ergometrine can also cause hypertension and should not be given to women with pre-eclampsia or essential hypertension. Instead, a continuous infusion of oxytocin should be used.

Obstetrics 11

A 39-year-old wife of a sailor in the Argentine Navy was admitted to the labour ward from a hotel, where the couple had been staying while on a visit to London to see relatives. She was complaining of the sudden onset of lower abdominal pain about 3 hours previously. The duration of her gestation was 32 weeks by certain dates, and the height of the uterine fundus was compatible with this.

She had had four previous pregnancies. The first, at the age of 19, was uncomplicated. The second had ended spontaneously at 20 weeks following the onset of severe lower abdominal pain and bleeding requiring blood transfusion. The next two pregnancies were normal apart from one episode of threatened preterm labour at 28 weeks.

On admission, her temperature was 36.6°C, her pulse rate 72 beats/minute and her blood pressure 150/90. Abdominal examination revealed a cephalic presentation, three-fifths palpable. The uterus was tender on the left side of the fundus. Palpable contractions were occurring every 3 minutes. Vaginal examination revealed a cervix 0.5 cm dilated, but still 2 cm long, and firm.

Cardiotocography was commenced, and initially the tracing was normal. However, 2 hours later, the fetal heart rate showed a baseline tachycardia of 170 beats/minute with some loss of baseline variability, and shallow late decelerations. The tocograph revealed contractions every 1–2 minutes. At this time a vaginal loss of about 30 ml of fresh blood became apparent. A repeat cervical assessment revealed no change in dilatation or effacement.

1. Suggest the probable aetiology of the fetal asphyxia.
2. What action would you take to resolve this situation?
3. Describe the haematological complications which may occur in this situation.
4. Why should this woman's urinary output be monitored closely?

1. By far the most likely diagnosis in this case is placental abruption. This woman has three predisposing features in her history: high parity, age over 35 years and previous antepartum haemorrhage. On examination, suggestive features were the raised blood pressure and uterine tenderness. The high level of clinical suspicion was confirmed by the development of excessively frequent uterine contractions, and the onset of vaginal bleeding.

   The probable causes of fetal asphyxia in placental abruption are impaired gas exchange secondary to disruption of large areas of the placenta, and excessively frequent contractions with persistently raised baseline tone. The relative importance of these two factors will vary from case to case. In addition, if the bleeding seriously reduces maternal blood volume, hypotension and reflex vasoconstriction will further reduce the fetal oxygen supply. The usual fetal response seen is a baseline tachycardia with late decelerations, but if the process is very acute, a progressive fetal bradycardia may be seen.

2. Early reported series of cases of placental abruption reported a fetal loss rate of up to 80%, but, with the advent of cardiotocography, diagnosis has been much improved in cases with little or no revealed blood loss, resulting in earlier recourse to caesarean section and greatly improved neonatal survival rates. In this case, caesarean section is clearly mandatory.

3. A major cause of mortality in abruption is the development of a consumptive coagulopathy secondary to fibrin consumption in the retroplacental clot. Release of fibrin degradation products into the circulation, together with low platelet and fibrinogen levels, exacerbates the bleeding which is already occurring. Clotting factors should be monitored closely, and serious deficiencies corrected with an infusion of fresh frozen plasma. Emptying the uterus of its contents is, however, the only way to reverse the consumptive process.

4. Placental abruption is often associated with acute oliguria or anuria. This is due to the so-called 'uterorenal reflex' and to maternal hypotension and hypovolaemia. The major priority in its correction is adequate blood transfusion (usually at least 1 litre, but much more may be needed) and maintenance of glomerular filtration rate by infusion of colloids (such as Hartmann's solution). Diuretics should only be used as a last resort, if central venous pressure monitoring shows a normal pressure level without adequate urinary output (at least 50 ml per hour).

   In the case described, an emergency caesarean section resulted in the delivery of a live female infant weighing 1.9 kg, with Apgar scores of 6 at 1 minute, 8 at 5 minutes and 10 at 10 minutes. There was approximately 600 ml of retroplacental clot, which had separated about 30% of the placental area.

Obstetrics 12

An English, non-smoking, Caucasian printer's assistant first presented to a gynaecologist at the age of 17 complaining of severe dysmenorrhoea. She had irregular menstrual cycles, occurring every 6–8 weeks. She was treated by forcible dilatation of the cervix (to Hegar size 10) under general anaesthesia. This produced a temporary improvement in her symptoms, but at the age of 19 the procedure had to be repeated (this time dilatation was to Hegar 14).

She then presented again, at the age of 28, complaining of involuntary primary infertility. She conceived after 2 months treatment with clomiphene, but miscarried at 20 weeks gestation. Nine months later she conceived once again following clomiphene therapy, but miscarried again, this time at 16 weeks.

Her third conception followed therapy with clomiphene, dexamethasone and HCG injections. A cervical suture was inserted at 12 weeks gestation, but at 21 weeks she was admitted with painful uterine contractions and spontaneous rupture of the membranes. The suture was removed and she miscarried within 12 hours.

Her fourth pregnancy was once again conceived following clomiphene therapy. A cervical suture was inserted at 12 weeks gestation. At 24 weeks, she was admitted with painful uterine contractions, which could be recorded on a tocograph trace, and which were occurring every 3 minutes. Speculum examination showed the cervix to be 3 cm dilated, with bulging but intact membranes. She was afebrile and the fetal heart was easily detected with a Doppler ultrasound machine.

1. Describe the likely pathology underlying her dysmenorrhoea.
2. Why is she miscarrying so frequently?
3. Outline a more modern approach to this type of dysmenorrhoea.
4. How would you evaluate the situation at the time of her most recent admission?
5. Discuss a possible therapy which would enable the pregnancy to continue until the baby was viable.

1. The irregular menstrual cycle, and the fact that she needed clomiphene in order to ovulate, suggests that this woman had dysmenorrhoea secondary to anovulatory cycles. Anovulation is common in adolescence, but also occurs in association with inadequate body weight (< 45 kg), or pathological conditions such as polycystic ovarian disease. Because proper corpus luteum function is not established in the luteal phase of non-ovulatory cycles, with consequent hormonal imbalance (particularly progesterone deficiency), endometrial shedding and uterine activity during the menstrual period are both abnormal. This produces an abnormal pattern of cervical dilatation as the menstruum passes, leading to pain. There may also be an abnormality in cervical compliance secondary to the hormone imbalance.

2. In the 1950s and 60s, a popular method of treating primary dysmenorrhoea was forcible dilatation of the cervix under general anaesthesia. This reduced the amount of stretching of the cervix required for the menstruum to pass and thus reduced pain during menstruation. However, in a significant number of cases, it led to cervical laxity or 'incompetence' during pregnancy, as illustrated so graphically in this case.

3. Modern approaches centre around medical therapy, either to correct the underlying pathology, e.g. by encouraging weight gain, or by modifying hormone patterns, e.g. by administering luteal phase progestogens, or the combined oral contraceptive pill. Prostaglandin synthetase inhibitors such as mefenamic acid (Ponstan) may also help by suppressing abnormal uterine activity.

4. When someone is admitted with both preterm labour, and a cervical suture in situ, careful examination should be carried out to exclude conditions such as infection, premature rupture of the membranes, or placental abruption, which would preclude further attempts at conservative therapy. The vagina should be inspected carefully for evidence of infection (reddening, foul smell, the presence of pus) and swabs taken for immediate culture. The pH of the vagina should be tested with nitrazine sticks (if they turn from orange to black, indicating a pH above 5, this is suggestive — but not conclusive — that the membranes are ruptured, allowing alkaline liquor into the vagina). If there is any suggestion of localised or systemic infection (maternal pyrexia, raised white count, tachycardia), the cervical suture should be removed and labour allowed to continue.

   The uterus should be palpated carefully for localised tenderness, suggesting the possibility of a concealed abruption. Uterine hypertonus, indicated on the tocograph as frequent (one every 1–2 mins), irregular contractions, is often associated with abruption. The presence of placental abruption is a contraindication to conservative therapy, as further massive bleeding may threaten the mother's life.

   A midstream or catheter urine specimen should be tested for protein and sent for culture, as a urinary tract infection may be associated with preterm labour.

5. Once the above pathologies have been excluded as far as possible, further treatment in the form of beta-2 sympathomimetic suppression of uterine contractions may be used (using drugs such as salbutamol or ritodrine). In the present case, two 50 μg bolus doses of salbutamol were given intravenously at 5-minute intervals. The abolition of uterine activity which ensued was maintained with a continuing intravenous infusion of 4 μg per min. It was given using a small, battery powered infusion pump, which could be carried by the patient herself. This is more effective than oral therapy, even when the latter is given at the recommended frequency of every 4 hours. In the case described, labour was suppressed successfully until 31 weeks, when recurring contractions and maternal distress necessitated removal of the suture. Within a few hours a healthy 1.4 kg male was delivered spontaneously per vaginam. Mother and baby subsequently did well.

Obstetrics 13

An English, Caucasian schoolgirl booked in her first pregnancy at the age of 16. The putative father was a motor mechanic.

She was unsure of the date of her last menstrual period, but on examination at booking the uterine size was consistent with a 14-week gestation. The fetal heart was easily heard with a portable Doppler ultrasound machine. An ultrasound scan showed a gestation by crown–rump length of approximately 13 weeks.

Booking investigations showed the mother to be 1.5 metres tall, and she weighed 48 kg. Her blood pressure was 120/70 mmHg. Her haemoglobin level was 14.5 g/dl, VDRL was negative, and the rubella antibody titre >1 in 32 with no IgM detectable (immune). She was A rhesus +ve with no antibodies.

She was seen again 4 weeks later, when she was 17 weeks by ultrasound scan. The uterine size had only enlarged a little, but the fetal heart was still heard with the Doppler ultrasound. A further scan at this visit showed a normal fetus but diminished liquor. Ultrasound gestation by BPD was now 16 weeks. She had not gained weight, but she felt generally well with no nausea or tiredness. A further ultrasound was booked for 20 weeks gestation.

However, she attended at 19.5 weeks worried that she had not yet felt any fetal movements. The fetal heart could not be heard with the portable Doppler machine, and an ultrasound scan confirmed that the fetus was dead.

1. List the commoner causes of intrauterine death at this gestation.
2. How would you manage the pregnancy?
3. What investigations would you perform?

1. The best way of classifying the causes of 2nd trimester intrauterine death is to consider (i) causes primarily affecting the fetus (ii) causes primarily affecting the mother and (iii) causes affecting both.

   (i) Primary fetal defects are largely congenital. Thus, a considerable number of these babies (approximately one-third) will have anatomical abnormalities, such as anencephaly, renal agenesis (Potter's syndrome) cardiovascular abnormality, or omphalocoele. A small proportion (approximately 5%) will have chromosomal abnormalities such as Down's syndrome, other trisomies, or Turner's syndrome (XO).

   (ii) Causes primarily affecting the mother are serious maternal disorders such as diabetes, chronic renal failure, or severe heart disease. These disorders interfere with normal fetomaternal symbiosis, either because of metabolic disturbance or reduced maternal blood flow.

   (iii) The commonest disorders affecting both mother and fetus are infections such as rubella, cytomegalovirus and toxoplasmosis. These probably account for about 10% of midtrimester deaths. Rather more important in numerical terms are the cases, such as the one described, where the normal response of the mother to pregnancy appears to be diminished, and the fetus suffers from prolonged intrauterine growth retardation. In these cases, a common and striking feature is a failure of maternal plasma volume expansion. This often leads to the finding of an unusually high Hb concentration at booking, as in this case (this finding will of course be masked if the mother has an iron-deficient anaemia). There is little or no dependent oedema and sometimes other symptoms of normal pregnancy (nausea, tiredness) are absent. Why this happens is obscure, but there is evidence that some cases may be immunological in origin (failure of development of normal maternal antibody to paternal antigens), while others may be associated with maternal malnutrition, particularly if the mother is underweight at the beginning of the pregnancy. Factors such as smoking may also contribute.

   Other causes of second trimester intrauterine death, in which the aetiology is unknown, include placental abruption, fetomaternal haemorrhage, cord complications and maternal trauma (these latter two are extremely rare).

2. There are two main reasons why these pregnancies are best terminated promptly. Firstly, there is the emotional distress of the mother, knowing she has a dead fetus within her. Secondly, after 3–4 weeks, coagulation disorders may occur secondary to increasing consumption of clotting factors by the conceptus.

   There are a number of techniques available for terminating pregnancies in the midtrimester. Nearly all use some form of prostaglandin, to which the uterus is much more sensitive than to oxytocin at this gestation. A very potent agent is gemeprost (16, 16-dimethyl-trans-delta-2 prostaglandin E_1 methyl ester), which can be administered by vaginal application. An alternative is extra-amniotic prostaglandin E_2, which is effective but more time-consuming to set up. It is occasionally necessary to add oxytocin at up to 40 mu/min.

3. Perhaps the single most important investigation to be performed after delivery is a careful examination of the fetus and placenta. Swabs should be sent for culture. If the parents agree, postmortem examination by a perinatal pathologist is invaluable. Culture of fetal cells (such as fibroblasts) may be possible, allowing chromosomal analysis. The mother should be screened by estimating haemoglobin concentration, blood group antibodies and blood urea and electrolytes. Thyroid function tests, serum aminotransferase estimation and an oral glucose tolerance test may also be performed where facilities are available. Urine should be sent for culture and protein estimation. Antibody titres to rubella, cytomegalovirus, toxoplasma, cocksackie B, and herpes simplex virus should be checked twice at 3-weekly intervals.

The 42-year-old wife of a hotel night porter had entered the UK from the Philippines 10 years previously. She was generally fit and had no significant past medical history.

At the age of 37 she had her first pregnancy, which ended in a 12-week spontaneous abortion. The following year she conceived again, and this time delivered a live male infant weighing 3.1 kg at 38 weeks gestation. Following the delivery, she had a postpartum haemorrhage and was transfused 2 units of blood.

In her next pregnancy, at the age of 42, she booked at 19 weeks of amenorrhoea. An ultrasound scan showed a fetus appropriately sized for this gestation. Amniocentesis to screen for Down's syndrome was discussed, but as she was Roman Catholic and would not accept termination she decided not to have this investigation. On examination she was noted to be 1.48 m tall with a weight of 54 kg. Her blood pressure was 120/70 mmHg.

Her pregnancy progressed uneventfully. At 36 weeks her haemoglobin concentration was 10.6 g/dl. She was admitted at just over 38 weeks gestation in spontaneous labour. On examination the cervix was found to be 8 cm dilated. Her labour progressed rapidly and 30 minutes later she was fully dilated. The second stage lasted only 15 minutes and resulted in the spontaneous delivery of a live female infant with Apgar scores of 8 at 1 minute and 10 at 5 minutes. The delivery was accompanied by a measured blood loss of 300 ml. She was given intramuscular syntometrine (5 units of oxytocin and 0.5 mg of ergometrine), which stopped the haemorrhage, but controlled cord traction failed to deliver the placenta. It was therefore decided to undertake manual removal of the placenta.

Examination in theatre, with the aid of general anaesthesia, revealed a constriction ring at the junction of the upper and lower segments of the uterus, above which was entrapped the placenta. The surgeon's hand could not readily be passed above the constriction and so he requested that the mother be given 2% halothane to relax the uterus. Shortly after the anaesthetist had complied with this request, the patient took a large breath and then spontaneous ventilation ceased. The carotid pulse was no longer palpable.

1. What is the most likely cause of the woman's sudden collapse?
2. What resuscitative measures should be taken?
3. What precautions should be taken before manual removal of the placenta is performed?

1. This woman's collapse was due to severe blood loss, compounded by the effects of deep anaesthesia. A measured loss of 300 ml at delivery usually indicates a total loss of at least 500 ml (the extra going onto the towels and swabs and thus escaping collection). In addition, with a retained placenta, blood collects in the uterus and is only evident at the time of uterine evacuation. The extent of blood loss into the uterus is limited by uterine tone. When the uterus contracts, not only do the 'living ligatures' of the myometrium close off the blood vessels passing through the uterine wall, but the raised intrauterine pressure helps to staunch the flow. When this woman was given halothane, the uterus relaxed, which not only allowed the surgeon to insert his hand, but allowed the uterus to bleed briskly once more. The bleeding was not obvious, because the internal volume of the uterus increased as it relaxed, thus allowing the blood to accumulate within it without being observed by the surgeon.

2. The mainstay of resuscitation in hypovolaemia is intravenous fluid replacement (preferably with blood). This woman was given 500 ml Hartmann's solution initially and while this was being given some plasma was made up. She was then given 1500 ml of plasma; by this time 2 units of blood had been obtained and were infused as rapidly as possible. She was also given 12 mg of betamethasone intravenously to combat shock. Sometimes inotropic drugs such as ephedrine, or even adrenaline, are necessary to restore circulation, but they were not needed in this case.

    These resuscitative measures rapidly restored the circulation. Postoperatively her haemoglobin was only 8 g/dl, indicating haemodilution; the full volume of fluid lost had been replaced but she was still short of red cells. Clotting studies were normal, as were an electrocardiogram and a chest X-ray.

3. Before performing a manual removal of placenta, the following steps should be taken:

(i) Crossmatch at least 2 units of blood. If there is persistent bleeding, crossmatch at least 4 and warn the haematologist that more might be needed.

(ii) Set up an intravenous infusion if one is not already in place.

(iii) Do nothing further until the blood is ready and the anaesthetist has arrived.

(iv) Before giving an anaesthetic (an epidural or spinal is satisfactory in many cases, but if there is persistent bleeding, a general anaesthetic is safer in case there is sudden collapse or a need for operative intervention), catheterise the bladder and perform a vaginal examination. The placenta may already have separated and be lying in the vagina, in which case it can be delivered and an anaesthetic avoided. *Do not do this before the blood and anaesthetist are available* — it may trigger uterine bleeding, in which case an anaesthetic and uterine exploration are still necessary.

Obstetrics 15

A 33-year-old housewife booked in her fourth pregnancy. She was married to a medical laboratory scientific officer. Her first pregnancy had been at the age of 26, and had appeared normal until she went into labour at 39 weeks gestation. A female infant was born spontaneously in good condition but weighed only 2.33 kg (approximately the 1st centile, weight for gestational age). Two years later she had an ectopic pregnancy requiring a salpingectomy and a blood transfusion. A further year later she was pregnant again, this time with an intrauterine gestation. Shared care was undertaken with the general practitioner. At 28 weeks gestation she was admitted as an emergency with an antepartum haemorrhage of about 100 ml. On examination the cervix was fully dilated. Artificial rupture of membranes revealed a shoulder presentation and so an emergency lower segment caesarean section was performed. The baby was extracted with difficulty and was in poor condition at birth. It weighed 1.2 kg but died 15 hours later. Postmortem revealed extensive hyaline membrane in the lungs, and haemorrhage into the cerebral ventricles.

In her fourth pregnancy she booked at 9 weeks gestation. She weighed 60 kg and was normotensive. She was seen every two weeks until 25 weeks gestation, when she was admitted to hospital for 'rest and observation'. Scans showed good fetal growth.

At 27 weeks gestation, she complained of a small amount of bleeding per vaginam, and some lower abdominal 'tightenings'. Vaginal examination showed the cervix to be 4 cm dilated, with bulging membranes.

1. Suggest a reason why this woman repeatedly had either growth retarded or preterm babies, and antepartum haemorrhages.
2. Why did the second baby have both intraventricular haemorrhages and extensive hyaline membrane disease?
3. Suggest further management.

1. The clinical history of this woman suggests recurrent failure of placentation. In a normal pregnancy, chorionic villi burrow out from the embedded blastocyst into the surrounding endometrium. At about 20–24 weeks gestation, the trophoblast extends down into the myometrium and invades the spiral arteries feeding the placental bed. This enlarges the arteries and effectively prevents them from responding to circulating vasoconstrictors, ensuring an adequate blood supply to the placenta at all times. In some women, the 'secondary wave of trophoblastic infiltration', as it is called, seems recurrently to be defective. The reason for this is not clear, but there are some pointers to an immunological basis for the problem. For example, each successive pregnancy may fare better than the previous one (improving immune response); and sometimes a change of partner dramatically changes the woman's reproductive performance (more effective antigen). Whatever the cause, the resulting 'placental insufficiency' can produce either fetal growth retardation, or premature separation of the placenta associated with antepartum haemorrhage and preterm labour.

2. Intrapartum asphyxia in the preterm infant is implicated in the aetiology of both hyaline membrane disease, and intraventricular haemorrhage. The type II pneumocytes in the lung, which produce surfactant, are very sensitive to hypoxia and are selectively damaged by intrapartum asphyxia. Similarly, the germinal matrix of the lateral cerebral ventricles is very susceptible to damage from hypoxia and is rendered more sensitive to vascular instability and trauma, both of which are likely to occur in preterm delivery.

3. There are a number of priorities in the further management of this case. Firstly, the presentation of the baby must be determined reliably, preferably by ultrasound scan. Any presentation other than cephalic favours delivery by repeat caesarean section. Secondly, fetal condition should be investigated by cardiotocography using an ultrasound transducer. Unless the fetal heart rate tracing obtained is completely normal, urgent caesarean section should be considered in all cases, even when the presentation is cephalic. In the case under discussion, the fetus was shown to be in breech presentation, with a normal cardiotocograph trace. A decision was therefore made to proceed to urgent caesarean section, which was performed through a midline incision, with a vertical anterior incision in the uterus. This approach aims to minimise the trauma to both baby and mother, which can easily occur when a preterm baby is pulled through a small incision in a poorly formed lower segment. It also speeds up the delivery and thus minimises asphyxia.

   In the present case, the baby weighed 1.2 kg and was in good condition at delivery. She made good progress, although prolonged ventilation via an endotracheal tube resulted in subglottic stenosis which subsequently required surgery for its correction.

Obstetrics 16

Mrs J H was a 23-year-old primigravida. She was employed as a clerical assistant by the local council and her husband was a chef.

She first attended the antenatal clinic for booking 16 weeks after her last menstrual period. She had an irregular menstrual cycle of 4–6 weeks. She had a history of depression and had also been investigated for possible thyrotoxicosis 4 years before the pregnancy. The only significant feature in her family history was that she had a nephew who was a juvenile-onset diabetic.

There was no abnormality on general examination. Abdominal palpation revealed that the uterine size was compatible with a pregnancy of 16 weeks duration. Routine urine analysis revealed 2% glycosuria, but no other abnormality. Because of this finding and the family history of diabetes a 75 g oral glucose tolerance test was performed. The result of this was (Table 3):

Table 3

Time	Glucose Level mmol/l (glucose oxidase method; venous plasma)
Fasting	6.5
30 min	10.6
1 h	14.9
1.5 h	17.8
2 h	16.8
2.5 h	15.4
3 h	10.2

1. Does this woman have gestational diabetes?
2. What further investigations would you perform on her?
3. How would you manage the remainder of her ante natal period?

1. Pregnancy imposes a stress on maternal carbohydrate metabolism which results in a two- to three-fold increase in fasting and postprandial plasma insulin concentrations. If the insulin secretory reserve of the pancreas is exceeded then diabetes mellitus results, usually in the second half of pregnancy when the stress is maximal. The impairment of glucose tolerance is frequently only minor, but a small number of women, of whom this patient is an example, develop frank diabetes with a fasting venous plasma glucose in excess of 6.0 mmol/l. The early onset of diabetes in this patient's pregnancy suggests that she may have had unrecognised glucose intolerance before becoming pregnant and that she may not have true 'gestational diabetes', a diagnosis which implies normal glucose tolerance in the non-pregnant state.

2. The plasma glucose concentrations observed after an oral glucose load are not representative of those which occur during a normal day. All patients with an abnormal glucose tolerance test should therefore be admitted to hospital for a series of plasma glucose estimations while consuming a diet appropriate for their build. A typical 'four-point profile' would comprise estimations taken before breakfast, lunch, tea and supper, e.g. 7 a.m., 12.00 midday, 5 p.m. and 9.30 p.m.; 1 hour postprandial values are also useful, particularly if there is persistent glycosuria.

3. The key to the successful management of diabetes in pregnancy is the achievement of maternal blood sugar levels as close to normal as possible. If there is only a slight disturbance of glucose homeostasis, dietary advice may be all that is required to achieve normoglycaemia. If, however, the preprandial values exceed 5.5 mmol/l and the postprandial values exceed 8.0 mmol/l then insulin therapy is indicated. The aim of treatment is to achieve pre- and postprandial plasma glucose concentrations of less than 5.0 and 7.0 mmol/l respectively. Whilst a single or twice-daily injection regime may be sufficient, even better control may be obtained by four times a day dosage (e.g. the novopen system).

   In the case described, the mean preprandial plasma glucose concentration was 6.8 mmol/l and that 2 hours postprandial was 8.9 mmol/l. Good control was achieved with a twice daily mixture of short and intermediate acting insulins.

   Although the current trend is to allow pregnancy in diabetic women to continue near to her due date, it is occasionally necessary to deliver the fetus before this. It is therefore important to be certain of the duration of pregnancy and, whenever possible, ultrasound measurements of the fetus should be obtained before 20 weeks gestation to confirm correct dating. Serial ultrasound measurements (particularly of the abdominal circumference) should subsequently be made to detect excessive fetal growth which may indicate poor control of the diabetes.

   The fetus of the diabetic mother is at increased risk of sudden intrauterine death in late pregnancy. Conventional methods of assessing fetal well being such as ultrasound biophysical profiles, doppler umbilical artery blood velocity waveform analysis, and fetal movement counting ('kick charts') have some value; antenatal cardiotocography can also be useful if any of these monitoring systems show an abnormality. At the present time, however, none of our monitoring systems will effectively predict sudden intrauterine death from a metabolic cause such as ketoacidosis or acute hypoglycaemia.

Provided there are no obstetric complications of pregnancy and diabetic control is satisfactory, there is no need to admit these patients to hospital. Adequate information about plasma glucose concentrations can be obtained at home using 'blood glucose sticks', ideally together with one or other of the meters that can be used to 'read' the colour change on the stick.

If good diabetic control has been achieved and there is no obstetric contraindication, the aim should be to achieve a vaginal delivery in the 39th week of pregnancy.

Obstetrics 17

An unmarried hairdresser became pregnant for the first time at the age of 20. She had a regular 28-day cycle and was certain of the date of her last menstrual period. She and her boyfriend had not been using any contraception. They were not living together; she shared a flat with two girlfriends and her boyfriend still lived at home with his divorced mother.

She first saw her family doctor when she was 16 weeks pregnant and asked to be delivered in the GP obstetric unit. The only significant medical history was that she smoked at least 20 cigarettes a day and had had a treated attack of gonorrhoea 2 years previously. As the pregnancy appeared to be progressing normally he agreed that she should remain under his care.

When she was 20 weeks pregnant, ++ proteinuria was detected on dipstick testing. A midstream urine (MSU) specimen was sent for bacteriology and amoxycillin was prescribed for a presumed urinary tract infection. The MSU did not contain protein and was sterile on culture. At about this time she attended the hospital's 'special clinic' because of vaginal discharge, dysuria and vulval soreness. She was generally unwell with 'flu-like symptoms and a low-grade fever. Examination revealed multiple small vesicular lesions and several exquisitely painful ulcers, up to 3 mm in diameter, on the inner aspect of the right labium minus. Viral culture confirmed the diagnosis of a herpes genitalis (herpes simplex virus type II) infection. She was treated with topical acyclovir and systemic amoxycillin. The GP was informed (with the patient's approval) of the infection. At 37 weeks she developed oedema of her ankles. At 38 weeks proteinuria was detected on routine urine testing once more, but was again absent from an MSU. Subsequent urine analysis was normal but her oedema increased and at 41 weeks her blood pressure was recorded at 160/90 mmHg, having been 120/70 at booking and subsequently never higher than 130/80 mmHg. She was therefore referred to a consultant obstetrician for advice about her management. On admission to hospital, she complained of a recurrence of vulval soreness at the site of her previous herpes attack.

1. Comment on this patient's antenatal care.
2. How would you manage her delivery?

1. A single, poorly supported woman who smokes and gives a history of previous genital infection is at substantially increased risk of both preterm delivery and intrauterine growth retardation. It would therefore have been wise for the general practitioner to involve the consultant obstetric team in her management from an early stage, preferably soon after booking.

   Herpes simplex virus type II is the commonest viral infection of the genital tract and its incidence appears to be increasing inexorably. Although the commonest presentation is an acute vulvitis with ulcerating vesicular lesions that cause dysuria and exquisite pain, nearly 50% of cases occur via an asymptomatic cervical infection. It is possible that the proteinuria detected during the antenatal visit preceding development of symptoms in this patient was due to a vaginal discharge resulting from herpetic cervicitis. Herpes simplex virus can have a profound effect on pregnancy outcome and the patient should have been referred to an obstetrician for further investigation after the diagnosis had been made. Spontaneous abortion follows early pregnancy infection in a third of primary cases and, although the virus does not usually cross the placenta, when this occurs it may cause severe congenital malformations including microcephaly, intracranial calcification, micro-ophthalmos and retinal dysplasia. Like herpes simplex virus type I, the type II virus remains dormant in infected nerve root ganglia and may be reactivated by a number of factors, including emotional stress.

2. The greatest risk for the fetus is infection at the time of delivery. Infection occurs in a significant proportion of babies born to women who have had a primary attack of herpes in the week preceding delivery and, of these, approximately half die or suffer serious neurological sequelae secondary to disseminated infection. Therefore, if a primary attack of herpes is suspected, swabs of the ulcers and from the cervix should be sent in viral transport medium for inoculation into human cell cultures to confirm the diagnosis. If the virus is present, typical cytopathic changes occur in 2–4 days.

   Caesarean section appears to reduce the risk of infection following a primary attack in late pregnancy, and is the preferred method of delivery if labour occurs when there is a likelihood of virus shedding (either on clinical grounds, or confirmed by culture), provided the fetal membranes are intact or within 4 hours of their spontaneous rupture. The situation in the case of a recurrent lesion is less clear, probably because the baby has substantial passive immunity from maternal antibodies transferred across the placenta. If the mother objects to caesarean section, then vaginal delivery and prophylactic treatment of the neonate with acyclovir would be considered reasonable by many. In the absence of clinical signs of a herpetic lesion, routine weekly viral culture of cervical swabs is no longer recommended. Instead, swabs should be taken from the baby at delivery, and the infant commenced on acyclovir if the culture is positive, or at the first signs of any systemic infection.

   This patient's blood pressure settled to 130/80 mmHg after her admission to hospital and vulval and cervical swabs were taken for herpes virus culture at this time. They proved positive and she was therefore delivered by elective lower segment caesarean section.

Obstetrics 18

A 24-year-old woman who booked with her family doctor for GP unit confinement was referred for consultant care at 17 weeks because of a twin pregnancy. This had been diagnosed during an ultrasound scan performed because of uncertain dates; she had become pregnant while taking a progestogen-only oral contraceptive. She had a 15-month-old son who had been delivered normally at 38 weeks and weighed 2.92 kg at birth. He had suffered unexplained cyanotic attacks after delivery and had been observed in the special care baby unit for 6 days, but his subsequent progress had been normal.

At booking (17 weeks by ultrasound) the symphy sis-fundal height was 22 cm. Prophylactic oral iron and folic acid were prescribed and further ultrasound scans were arranged at 28, 32 and 36 weeks to assess fetal growth.

At 28 weeks the symphysis–fundal height was only 30 cm and the ultrasound measurements showed both fetuses to be small for dates, one slightly growth retarded (size equivalent to the mean for 26–27 weeks), the other grossly so (size equivalent to the mean for 22–23 weeks).

She was therefore admitted for further investigation. During the next 8 weeks ultrasound measurements were made at fortnightly intervals. Cardiotocography was performed on each fetus, initially on alternate days and subsequently on a daily basis.

The head and abdomen circumference measurements confirmed symmetrical growth retardation of both of the twins until 34 weeks, when the head growth of the smaller twin appeared to cease while its abdominal girth continued to enlarge. The volume of the amniotic fluid surrounding the smaller fetus was noted to be reduced, while that surrounding the larger fetus, whose head was engaged in the pelvis, appeared normal in amount. The patient herself remained well. She had a blood pressure of 110/70–120/80 and urine analysis was normal.

1. What are the possible explanations for the clinical findings?
2. How would you manage the remainder of this pregnancy?

1. Despite the fact that multiple pregnancy is characterised by exaggerated physiological changes, e.g. enhanced plasma expansion, twin fetuses rarely achieve their full growth potential and ultrasound measurements frequently reveal a slowing of growth, particularly during the third trimester of pregnancy. In this case, the measurements of the larger twin appear to reflect this pattern. The measurements of the smaller twin are not, however, typical of twin gestation and suggest a more sinister underlying pathology.

   Superfetation (fertilisation of two ova released at different times) has never been demonstrated in human pregnancy and can be excluded because of the similar measurements of the two fetuses at 14 weeks. Infective causes of severe growth retardation, e.g. congenital rubella syndrome, cytomegalovirus, or toxoplasmosis cannot be excluded, but were thought to be unlikely as only one fetus appeared affected. The cessation of head growth in the smaller fetus, with continued enlargement of the trunk is suggestive of microcephaly (which can be due to cytomegalovirus infection, but is usually of unknown cause).

   Some relatively common chromosomal abnormalities such as trisomy 21 (Down's syndrome), trisomy 18 (Edward's syndrome), or Turner's syndrome (45 XO) may be associated with impaired cranial growth. In addition, certain rare chromosomal deletion defects, such as the deletion of the short arm of chromosome 5 (5 p-) (the Cri du chat syndrome) and the deletion of the long arm of chromosome 13 (13q-) usually cause overt microcephaly.

2. The possibility that the severe growth retardation of the smaller twin was due to a potentially lethal congenital abnormality was a source of anxiety in managing this case. It was decided, however, to assume that the twin was in fact normal, and rely on the patient's assessment of fetal movements and the daily cardiotocographic (CTG) recordings obtained from each fetus, to assess the well-being of the babies. Delivery was to be undertaken as an emergency if any of these parameters became abnormal, or electively at the 37th week of pregnancy, whichever came first. Although both fetuses remained active, the CTG of the smaller twin began to show reduced baseline variability and occasional early decelerations at 36 weeks. The cervix was favourable, but because it was felt that the smaller twin would not tolerate the stress of labour, an elective caesarean section was performed.

   Both infants were male and weighed 2.16 and 1.63 kg respectively. The cause in the disparity between their birthweights was immediately apparent, as the larger twin was clinically plethoric and on investigation was shown to be polycythaemic with a haemoglobin of 23 g/dl and a packed cell volume of 82%. The smaller twin was clinically anaemic and had a haemoglobin of 11 g/dl and a packed cell volume of 15%.

   Clinical examination of the placenta (subsequently confirmed by histological examination) revealed two amniotic sacs and a single chorionic layer. The twin transfusion syndrome evident in this case therefore appears to explain the severe growth retardation of one twin. This is a rare complication of twin pregnancy and in its most florid form may present in the second trimester with polyhydramnios in one sac and oligohydramnios in the other. Premature labour, usually early in the third trimester, frequently occurs in this situation. When the syndrome is suspected, as in this case, from the ultrasound findings, frequent non-stressed cardiotocographic tracings appear to be the most sensitive test for determining the optimal time for delivery.

Obstetrics 19

A 21-year-old garage secretary booked for antenatal care at 12 weeks. She had had two previous pregnancies, 2 and 5 years earlier. Both pregnancies had been terminated at approximately 8 weeks for social reasons. She had used oral contraception after the first termination but had stopped after 4 years because of weight gain. She and her partner subsequently used a sheath for contraception and the second pregnancy resulted from a failure of this method. Shortly after the second termination they married and the present pregnancy had been planned. Her menarche had occurred at the age of 11 years and menstruation, which occurred every 28 days, lasted for 4–5 days. Her past history included a meniscectomy and an episode of cystitis. She smoked 2 cigarettes a day. At the time she conceived she had been attending a swimming club and had put herself on a 1000 calorie reducing diet.

On examination she was 170 cm tall and weighed 96 kg. Her blood pressure was 125/75 mmHg. She was obese, but there was no other abnormality on general examination. Pelvic examination confirmed the uterine size to be compatible with 12 weeks gestation. There was no abnormality of the vulva, vagina, cervix or adnexa.

1. What effect does obesity have on pregnancy?
2. What dietary advice would you give this patient?

1. Obesity is an easily recognisable maternal high-risk factor. Hypertension is diagnosed more commonly in the pregnant woman who is overweight and the incidence increases with the degree of obesity. This is partly due to the fact that blood pressure measurements are usually taken in these patients using a standard adult cuff, which is inappropriately small for the arm circumference of obese individuals. It is, however, also due to the effect of obesity on the maternal cardiovascular system. It is therefore important always to measure the blood pressure of obese individuals with a large cuff.

   Both obesity and pregnancy impose a stress on the insulin-producing beta-cells of the pancreatic islets of Langerhans. Significant maternal glucose intolerance (gestational diabetes) is approximately 5 times more frequent in overweight women, and 50% of women with gestational diabetes are obese. Even though most obese pregnant women have normal glucose tolerance, their infants are heavier (and fatter) than those of non-obese subjects; they are 4 times more likely to have macrosomic infants (>4 kg) than women of normal weight. It is therefore not surprising that many studies have shown a significant increase in prolonged labour, assisted vaginal deliveries and caesarean sections for cephalopelvic disproportion in these women. On the other hand, prematurity and intrauterine growth retardation are half as common in obese women compared to those who are non-obese. Some studies have shown an increased perinatal mortality in association with maternal obesity. This appears to result from traumatic vaginal delivery and no difference in perinatal outcome has been observed in more recent studies with earlier recourse to caesarean section.

2. The average weight gain during pregnancy is 12.5 kg. Approximately 4 kg of this is storage fat, largely deposited in the first two-thirds of pregnancy. At the time of conception, at least 20% of the body composition is storage fat and in an obese woman fat may account for more than 50% of body weight. It is therefore illogical for an obese woman to gain as much fat during pregnancy as a lean woman of similar height. An average pregnancy weight gain of 7–9 kg therefore appears appropriate for the patient with obesity preceding pregnancy. This weight gain has been shown to be associated with an optimal perinatal outcome in obese patients. The dietary advice that should be given to prevent unnecessary additional fat accumulation has to be tailored to the individual patient, but usually involves a balanced nutrient intake containing 1500-1800 calories. Such a diet has been shown to reduce the stress on the pancreatic B-cell in obese women and does not have any unfavourable effects on neonatal outcome.

Obstetrics 20

A 23-year-old shop assistant was referred to the antenatal clinic for booking. She had been married for 4 years to a tool fitter and was pregnant for the first time. She had stopped using the combined oral contraceptive 3 months earlier and was uncertain of the date of her last menstrual period, but thought she was about 12 weeks pregnant. She had not experienced any pain or vaginal bleeding since her last period. Her only significant past medical history was an episode of cystitis, treated with antibiotics, the previous year. She had never had any operations and was not taking any medication. There was no relevant family history.

General examination showed her to be a fit woman with a normal temperature. Her blood pressure was 125/75 mmHg and her pulse 84 beats/minute. Her breasts were firm. Abdominal palpation revealed a firm mass arising from the pelvis. This was equivalent in size to a 16 weeks pregnant uterus and was lying to the left of the midline. There was a small viral wart on the left of her vulva which was otherwise normal. Her vagina and cervix were also normal. Because she was very tense, the uterine size was difficult to assess. However, it appeared to be equivalent to an 8–10 weeks gestation and it was retroverted. Apparently inseparable from it was a mass of approximately 12 cm diameter. This had a smooth, regular outline but was of limited mobility. The following investigations were performed (Table 4) :

Table 4

Urine analysis	normal
Pregnancy test	positive
Haemoglobin	12.7 g/dl
White cell count	12.2 x 10^9/l
Differential:	
Polymorphs	79%
Lymphocytes	16%
Monocytes	4%
Eosinophils	1%
The film confirmed a 'mild neutrophilia'	
Cervical smear	negative
Midstream urine	no growth
	normal microscopy

All other routine booking investigations were normal.

1. Give a differential diagnosis.
2. What investigations would you perform to clarify the diagnosis?
3. How would you manage the two most likely causes?

1. The most likely diagnoses are an ovarian neoplasm or a uterine fibroid associated with a normal intrauterine pregnancy.

   At first sight, the raised white cell count and neutrophil leucocytosis suggest an inflammatory cause, but a rise in the total white cell count, due mainly to an increase in neutrophils, is physiological in pregnancy. A figure of 12.2 x 10^9/l is higher than average in the first trimester, but is within the normal range.

   Functional ovarian tumours (e.g. a corpus luteum cyst) are relatively common in pregnancy but rarely exceed 6–8 cm in diameter and are normally fluctuant. The possibility of an extrauterine pregnancy cannot be excluded. A tubal pregnancy this large is unlikely, but an ovarian or a secondary abdominal pregnancy may reach this size. A hydrosalpinx is rarely this big; it would, in any case, appear cystic and probably be associated with infertility. A pyosalpinx or pelvic abscess can also be excluded in a patient who is afebrile and pain free. A broad ligament cyst is a remote possibility, but as the mass in this case felt firm the diagnosis seems unlikely. Pregnancy in one horn of a bicornuate uterus is rare but cannot be excluded on the clinical history presented. A pelvic kidney would not be this large. Endometriosis with ovarian involvement is a possibility, but would almost certainly present with pain and is also likely to cause infertility.

2. An ultrasound scan, after getting the patient to fill her bladder, should clarify the diagnosis. Laparoscopy is contraindicated with a mass of this size. Laparotomy may, however, prove to be necessary.

   During pregnancy, the blood flow to uterine fibroids increases causing them to grow. This may result in compression of the blood vessels supplying the fibroid and result in infarction or 'red degeneration'. Despite this, no attempt should be made to perform a myomectomy in a pregnant patient. Apart from the probable disruption of the pregnancy, such surgery is fraught with complications, in particular uncontrollable haemorrhage that may necessitate hysterectomy.

   The ultrasound scan demonstrated that this patient had a 10-cm diameter semisolid ovarian neoplasm and a normal 12-week intrauterine pregnancy. Ovarian tumours are diagnosed in approximately 1:1000 pregnancies, usually at the first antenatal visit. Only 2–3% of such tumours are likely to be malignant, but they should always be removed because complications such as torsion, rupture and haemorrhage are more common in pregnancy. In addition, when impacted in the pelvis, they predispose to an unstable lie and may cause obstructed labour. Small ovarian cysts (less than 6 cm diameter) diagnosed during the first trimester are likely to be corpus luteum cysts. If the patient is asymptomatic she should be rescanned at approximately 12–14 weeks. If the cyst persists, then a laparotomy is indicated at this time. Any cyst larger than 6 cm and any solid or semisolid neoplasm is an indication for laparotomy as early as possible in the second trimester. Occasionally, a pedunculated subserous fibroid will be confused on ultrasound with a solid ovarian tumour and the error only discovered at laparotomy. No attempt should be made to remove such fibroids. Asymptomatic ovarian tumours are seldom recognised in the third trimester and any that are, are best removed after delivery.

This patient had a laparotomy and left salpingo-oophorectomy at 14 weeks. The ovary was enlarged by a dermoid cyst (benign teratoma), which is the commonest ovarian tumour at this age and accounts for nearly 20% of all ovarian neoplasms.

Obstetrics 21

A 35-year-old married shop assistant was referred as an emergency for antenatal assessment because of intractable vomiting. She had been taking a combined oral contraceptive pill for 4 years but 3 months earlier had forgotten to take it on 2 successive nights and subsequently missed a withdrawal bleed. Her suspicion that she might be pregnant increased when she developed breast tenderness and vomiting. Although a pregnancy test confirmed her worst fears, she and her husband had reconciled themselves to the fact that their 15-year-old son and 13-year-old daughter were to be joined by a baby brother or sister. Her first pregnancy, a breech delivery, had been complicated by marked nausea and sickness and she was therefore not surprised when this persisted. Her second pregnancy had, however, been entirely normal.

The vomiting initially occurred only in the morning, but as the pregnancy progressed it occurred throughout the day and became progressively more severe. During the 48 hours prior to her admission she had been unable to retain even clear fluids and had sought the assistance of her family doctor. He had been concerned at her general condition and the fact that her uterus appeared to be at least 4 weeks larger than the duration of pregnancy, calculated from the date of her last pill withdrawal bleed. She had not experienced any other vaginal bleeding nor any pain since this time. There had been no change in her bowel habit and she had no urinary symptoms. Apart from an appendicectomy at the age of 21 years her past history was unremarkable. There was no relevant family history.

On examination she was clearly dehydrated and distressed by her constant nausea and persistent vomiting. Her temperature was 36.8°C, pulse rate 104 beats/minute and blood pressure 100/60 mmHg. She did not appear anaemic and there was no other abnormality on general examination. Her breasts were normal. Abdominal palpation revealed a 16-week size uterus, which was regular in outline. There was no other suggestion of abdominal distension and her abdomen was non-tender with normal bowel sounds. Vaginal examination was normal and bimanual palpation confirmed the uterine size. A pregnancy test was strongly positive.

1. What is the differential diagnosis?
2. What investigations would you perform?
3. What are the complications of this condition?
4. Name a well-known authoress who died of this condition.

1. The patient has hyperemesis gravidarum and uncertain dates. If it is assumed that she became pregnant during the month she missed her oral contraceptive pills, then her uterus is about 4 weeks larger than expected. Multiple pregnancy and hydatidiform mole, both of which predispose to hyperemesis in pregnancy, must therefore be excluded. This can be done most easily by ultrasound scanning. The number of fetuses present can be counted and the gestation assessed by measurement of the biparietal diameter. With appropriate ultrasound intensity (low gain), an absence of fetal parts and a classical 'snow storm appearance' will confirm a hydatidiform mole. A pregnancy test on an 'early morning' urine specimen which is positive at 1:200 is also strongly suggestive of a hydatidiform mole.

   Gastroenteritis, hepatitis, cholecystitis, hiatus hernia, peptic ulcer and intestinal obstruction may all be mimicked by hyperemesis but can be excluded on clinical grounds in this case.

2. Blood should be sent for plasma electrolytes, blood urea estimation and liver function tests. A full blood count should also be obtained.

   The patient should be nursed in a quiet single room, with no oral intake allowed, apart from occasional sips of water. Rehydration should be achieved by giving intravenous fluids and nausea and vomiting quelled using antiemetics.

   While awaiting the urea and electrolyte results, an intravenous infusion of dextrose saline BP should be commenced. Potassium supplements should be added to the infusion fluid when the plasma electrolyte concentrations are known. A careful fluid balance record must be maintained and the patient should be weighed daily. Suitable antiemetics include promethazine, 25–50 mg, or chlorpromazine, 25–50 mg, by intramuscular injection every 4–6 hours as required. These drugs cause drowsiness and may produce a dry mouth. Other drugs that are used include promazine and perphenazine. All these drugs, especially the last, may cause extrapyramidal neurological effects such as oculogyric crises. Vitamin C, vitamin B complex and vitamin B6 (pyridoxine) may be added to the infusion fluids if there has been prolonged starvation. Although there is no proven cause for hyperemesis, many of these women have emotional problems. Psychiatric consultation may be necessary and isolation from domestic stress and relatives may be beneficial.

   When the patient has stopped vomiting for 24–48 hours and has both a normal urine output and normal plasma electrolytes, oral fluid intake should be increased to 50 ml hourly. If this is tolerated she should be given easily digested high-energy foods (e.g. milk, fruit juices, etc.) frequently, in small amounts. If these are tolerated, the diet should progress to semisolid foods (e.g. boiled eggs, cereal, etc.).

   When the patient has returned to her normal diet and activity she should be discharged home on oral antiemetic therapy. She should be advised not to drive or operate machinery while taking antiemetic drugs. Considerable anxiety has been expressed about the possible teratogenic effects of antiemetics. Extensive studies in Britain and the United States of America have exonerated these preparations and demonstrated their safety during pregnancy.

3. Rare complications of persistent vomiting include rupture of the oesophagus, aspiration pneumonitis, haemorrhagic retiniitis and dental erosion.

4. Maternal death from hyperemesis is recorded (Charlotte Bronte succumbed to the disorder), but it is now rare and once treated there is no apparent effect on the pregnancy.

The ultrasound scan in this patient showed a normal 12-week pregnancy and her hyperemesis resolved rapidly with the therapy described.

Obstetrics 22

Mrs RA, a 36-year-old Saudi Arabian woman, was referred for antenatal booking by a consultant cardiologist. She had no idea of the date of her last period, but thought that she was about 5 months pregnant. This was her eleventh pregnancy following ten normal deliveries, all at home. Five children had died in infancy and 1 in the neonatal period. The cause of these deaths was unknown. Her last and youngest child was 3 years old.

Nine months earlier Mrs RA had been admitted to hospital in acute congestive cardiac failure. A diagnosis of mitral stenosis and incompetence due to rheumatic heart disease was made and she was treated with digoxin and diuretics. She had subsequently remained well and while awaiting cardiac catheterisation and possible valve replacement she became pregnant. She denied any shortage of breath at rest and appeared to have normal exercise tolerance. There was no other past obstetric, medical or family history. She was taking oral digoxin 0.25 mg, frusemide 40 mg, phenoxymethyl penicillin 250 mg daily and oral potassium supplements twice daily.

She appeared underweight (46 kg) for her height (155 cm), but was not anaemic and there was no abnormality on general examination. Her jugular venous pressure appeared normal and there was no clubbing. Her pulse rate was 76 beats/minute and was irregular. On auscultation her apex rate was 86 beats/minute with a loud pansystolic murmur. There was also a midsystolic murmur in the mitral area. An exaggerated second heart sound was heard in the pulmonary area. Marked cardiomegaly and a left parasternal heave were apparent. There were no adventitious sounds with respiration. Abdominal palpation revealed the uterine size to be compatible with 20 weeks gestation and this was confirmed by ultrasound measurement of the fetal biparietal diameter. There was no abnormality on pelvic examination. An echocardiogram was performed. This confirmed that she had atrial fibrillation and that there was 'severe calcification of the mitral valve with gross enlargement of the left atrium and left ventricle and probably some enlargement of the right ventricle'.

1. Describe the physiological changes in cardiac dynamics that occur during pregnancy.
2. How would you manage the remainder of this patient's pregnancy?
3. Describe the management of her labour.
4. What contraception would you advise for her?

1. Pregnancy is associated with a rise in cardiac output of approximately 30–40%. This occurs progressively as gestation advances, but the greatest increase takes place in the first and second trimesters and is then maintained to delivery. The increase in cardiac output results both from an increase in stroke volume and a rise in the maternal heart rate of 10–15 beats per minute. In labour cardiac output rises by a further 25%. Cardiac output is very sensitive to posture during pregnancy. This is largely due to interference with venous return resulting from compression of the inferior vena cava by the pregnant uterus. Turning a patient from the supine to the left lateral position may increase the cardiac output by as much as 25%.

2. All pregnant women with significant cardiac disease should be seen by a cardiologist and an obstetrician fortnightly until 30 weeks and then weekly thereafter. Patients with a history of previous cardiac failure should be admitted for rest from 34–36 weeks until delivery. Women with less severe disease may continue as outpatients provided they can obtain adequate rest at home. Any patient who develops symptoms or signs of heart failure should be admitted. At each clinic visit, the woman must be carefully examined and this examination must include pulse rate, apex rate, auscultation of the heart and lungs (particularly the bases posteriorly), and assessment of the jugular venous pressure and peripheral oedema. All findings must be carefully recorded, as should any complaints of shortness of breath at night (paroxysmal nocturnal dyspnoea).

   Closed mitral valvotomy was considered in this patient, but was considered inappropriate because of the evidence of mitral incompetence. Open heart surgery is contraindicated because of the high associated fetal mortality.

   Fetal growth should be monitored with ultrasound. If there is any ultrasound or clinical suggestion of intrauterine growth retardation, fetal well-being should be assessed with antenatal cardiotocography and consideration given to early delivery.

3. Spontaneous vaginal delivery with epidural anaesthesia to remove the stress (and resulting maternal tachycardia) resulting from labour pain, is the ideal mode of delivery. An experienced anaesthetist is vital, as acute hypotension should be avoided, as should fluid overload. Maternal bearing down should be kept to a minimum and, in cases of severe disease, elective instrumental delivery is probably preferable. If induction of labour is necessary, then consideration should be given to using repeated low dose (1 mg) prostaglandin E_2 to minimise the risk of failed induction if the cervix is unfavourable. Caesarean section should be avoided if possible because the physical stress on the mother is increased and there is also a risk of subacute bacterial endocarditis (SBE) if wound infection occurs. Should augmentation of labour be necessary, oxytocin should be administered using a syringe pump to minimise the volume of fluid infused. A careful fluid balance record must be maintained because oxytocin has an antidiuretic action even in low doses.

   The patient should labour in a semisitting position. If the lithotomy position is used for an instrumental delivery, lateral tilt or wedging is important to prevent postural hypotension. Broad-spectrum antibiotics, such as amoxycillin or a cephalosporin, should be given by parenteral injection during labour and continued orally for 5 days after delivery to minimise the risk of SBE. (Some authorities recommend the more potent combination of penicillin and gentamycin.) Continuous fetal heart rate monitoring should be performed during labour.

The greatest risk of cardiac failure occurs during, and immediately after, delivery. Drugs and equipment necessary to treat acute cardiac failure should therefore be immediately to hand.

Ergometrine should not be given in the third stage of labour as this may cause a rapid increase in central venous pressure and lead to cardiac failure. Most obstetricians prefer to avoid oxytocics, but if a postpartum haemorrhage occurs, then an intravenous bolus of 5 units of oxytocin is acceptable.

4. This patient should be advised that sterilisation would be in her best interests. Contraception for the cardiac patient who does not wish to be sterilised is difficult, since combined oestrogen-progestogen oral contraceptives predispose to fluid retention, hyperlipidaemia and venous thromboembolism. The intrauterine device may be associated with infection, both pelvic and valvular. Barrier methods have a much higher failure rate and this lessens their value for such patients. Progestogen-only contraception (the 'minipill') probably represents the best compromise, if sterilisation is unacceptable.

Obstetrics 23

A 22-year-old clerk, married to a carpenter, was first seen at 17 weeks gestation in her third pregnancy. Her first two pregnancies had ended as miscarriages, 1 and 2 years earlier, at 11 and 14 weeks gestation respectively. At booking she complained that she had been troubled by intermittent headaches for several weeks. On examination her blood pressure was noted to be 160/110 mmHg. She had been treated for cystitis in the previous year, but had no other significant past medical or family history. She had used oral contraception for 11 months after her marriage at the age of 17 years. Her blood pressure had been normal while she was taking the pill. She was not taking any drugs and was not aware of any allergies.

There was no abnormality on general examination, apart from her elevated blood pressure. The only retinal changes were minimal a-v nipping and slight 'silver wiring'. Abdominal and pelvic examination revealed a 16-week size uterus. Because of her hypertension she was admitted for further investigation. All her booking investigations were normal, including her blood urea and uric acid. A 24-hour urine collection was made to assess her creatinine clearance and urinary vanillyl mandelic acid (VMA) excretion. Her creatinine clearance was normal, but to the surprise of all concerned the urinary VMA concentration was grossly elevated. A tentative diagnosis of a phaeochromocytoma was made and blood was taken for plasma noradrenaline measurement. This was 100 times the upper limit of normal, which is diagnostic of a phaeochromocytoma. Treatment with alpha-adrenergic and beta-adrenergic blocking drugs (phenoxybenzamine 10 mg t.i.d. and propranolol 40 g t.i.d.) was therefore started. A rapid decline in her blood pressure to normal levels occurred and was associated with cessation of her headaches.

1. What is a phaeochromocytoma?
2. How would you manage the rest of this pregnancy?

1. Phaechromocytoma is a catecholamine-producing tumour that arises from the chromaffin cells of the sympathoadrenal system, usually in the adrenal gland, but also along the sympathetic nervous chain, sometimes to aberrant and multiple locations. Approximately 8% are malignant and 10% are bilateral.

   Phaeochromocytoma accounts for only 0.1–0.5% of *all* causes of hypertension and is exceedingly rare in pregnancy. Despite its rarity it is, however, important because it is a consistent cause of maternal death. The diagnosis is unfortunately very easy to miss because many of the classical symptoms and signs of the condition occur frequently as normal symptoms of pregnancy, notably sweating, flushes, palpitations, headache and hypertension. Even when the diagnosis is made in the pregnant woman, the maternal and fetal mortality approach 50%. Clearly it is not possible to investigate every woman with these symptoms who has a rise in blood pressure during pregnancy. However, when hypertension occurs during early pregnancy and is episodic in nature, or related to posture, a phaeochromocytoma must be excluded. Catecholamines may produce glucose intolerance, so any patient with hypertension and glycosuria should also be investigated. The simplest investigation involves measurement of the catecholamine excretory product, vanillyl mandelic acid (VMA) in a 24-hour urine specimen — values in excess of 35 umol/24 hours are usually diagnostic. The result may be unreliable if the woman is on certain hypotensive drugs such as bethanidine and debrisoquine when the measurement is made, since these drugs may give falsely low VMA values. Fortunately, these particular drugs are seldom used in pregnant women. Measurement of plasma noradrenaline is specific, but single measurements may occasionally give false negative results if catecholamine release from the tumour only occurs intermittently.

   Surprisingly high levels of plasma noradrenaline may be obtained if blood sampling is performed in a patient who is under stress. Although this is unlikely to result in the mistaken diagnosis of phaeochromocytoma, venous blood samples should ideally be collected only when the patient has been resting in the semirecumbent position for an hour. The 'phentolamine blocking test' is potentially hazardous and is now obsolete.

   Localisation of the tumour usually involves X-ray techniques such as intravenous pyelography, arteriography and computed axial tomography, which cannot be used in pregnancy. However, ultrasound scanning is safe in pregnancy and its use in this case revealed a 'rounded homogeneous mass 3.5 cm in diameter lying adjacent to the upper pole of the right kidney'.

2. The alpha-blocker phenoxybenzamine is currently the drug of choice for treatment of phaeochromocytoma in pregnancy. It does not appear to have any adverse effect on the fetus. Use of beta-blockers such as propranolol is more controversial. In theory, they predispose to premature labour and intrauterine growth retardation and may reduce the fetal cardiac response to stress; in practice, they minimise the risk of maternal cardiac arrhythmias and probably have little adverse effect on a healthy fetus.

   A glucose tolerance test should be performed because of the

possibility that mild carbohydrate intolerance may occur. The infants delivered by these women are usually heavier than average and mild chemical diabetes may be a causal factor. Unnecessary abdominal palpation should be avoided as mechanical stimulation of the tumour may cause catecholamine release. The optimum time for delivery is a matter for debate. It is probably sensible to deliver the infant as soon as maturity can be assured, i.e. after 37–38 weeks gestation.

The available data suggest that labour is best avoided and that caesarean section is associated with a better maternal outcome. Anaesthesia in these patients is difficult. Sufficient sedation must be achieved to prevent catecholamine release from the tumour in response to anxiety over the operation. It is, however, also necessary to ensure that the baby is not unduly depressed at delivery. Atropine must be avoided as it produces a tachycardia and may elevate the blood pressure. A combination of sodium thiopentone, nitrous oxide, oxygen, succinyl suxamethonium and tubocurarine is usual. Morphine and pethidine should not be given, the former because it releases histamine, which in turn causes catecholamine release, and the latter because it may cause hypotension.

If the tumour has been located during pregnancy, as in this case, it is probably best to remove it immediately after caesarean section. This simplifies the postoperative management and avoids the risks associated with a second anaesthetic.

Obstetrics 24

A grand multiparous Bedouin woman, who was 34 years old, attended the antenatal clinic for the first time after approximately 8 months amenorrhoea. This was her ninth pregnancy. She had 7 children of whom the eldest was 17 and the youngest 2 years old. The first 6 children had all been born normally at home, but the last, a breech, had been delivered in hospital. She had also had 1 first trimester miscarriage. Before conception her menstrual cycle had been regular and she had not used any contraception for at least 2 years. There was no significant past medical or family history.

On examination she was obese (weight 78.5 kg; height 156 cm), but otherwise appeared healthy. Her blood pressure was 120/75 mmHg. Her breasts showed the usual changes associated with pregnancy. Her abdomen was distended and palpation confirmed a pregnant uterus. The fundal height and fetal size were compatible with 36 weeks gestation. There was marked hydramnios which made fetal palpation difficult. The lie was longitudinal with a cephalic presentation. The head was lying over the pelvic inlet but was freely mobile. Pelvic examination revealed an average size pelvis of normal shape. All booking investigations were normal.

1. What is a grand multipara and what is the significance of this descriptive term?
2. How would you establish the duration of pregnancy in this patient?
3. List five causes of hydramnios.

1. A woman who has delivered four children and is in her fifth pregnancy is known as a 'grand multipara'. Such women are more likely to experience both medical and obstetric problems, for example vascular disorders (especially hypertension), renal problems and gestational diabetes. It is likely that these problems are at least in part due to the fact that grand multiparae are usually older than the average pregnant woman. Repeated pregnancies may cause depletion of iron stores with consequent anaemia.

    Both pre-eclampsia and abruptio placentae are more common if there is pre-existing hypertension, which probably accounts for the increase in these conditions in grand multiparae.

    For reasons that are not clear the uteri of many of these women appear to be more relaxed than those of women of lower parity. This is associated with an increased amniotic fluid volume (polyhydramnios), and often results in an unstable lie with a variety of fetal malpresentations.

    Placenta praevia is two to four times more common in grand multiparae. It has been suggested that this is due to endometrial atrophy caused by repeated pregnancies. There is, however, no evidence for this rather implausible hypothesis. Congenital anomalies are also more common, due to an age-related increase in chromosomal abnormalities.

    Women become more obese with advancing age and the incidence of infants weighing more than 4 kg is increased (to about 20%). This can result in unexpected cephalopelvic disproportion and shoulder dystocia in women with hitherto normal obstetric histories. This possibility must always be borne in mind when cervical dilatation stops in the active phase of the first stage of labour in the grand multipara (i.e. when the cervix is fully effaced and 3 cm or more dilated). Injudicious use of an intravenous oxytocin infusion in such patients may result in uterine rupture.

    The incidence of primary postpartum haemorrhage is also increased in grand multiparae. It has been suggested that this is due to increased collagen deposition in the myometrium, resulting in reduced uterine contractility. This concept, has, however, been disputed.

    Late engagement of the fetal head, coupled with polyhydramnios, increases the frequency of cord presentation and prolapse.

    The rapid (precipitate) labour which may occur in these women can cause trauma, especially to the premature fetus, because of sudden compression and decompression of its head.

2. It is not possible to determine the duration of pregnancy accurately in the third trimester, especially near term. Ultrasound measurement of the fetal biparietal diameter will predict the duration of gestation to ± 10 days before 26 weeks, but in the third trimester this figure increases progressively to ± 3 weeks or more. Fetal X-rays are of limited value. The presence of a lower femoral epiphysis on an oblique AP X-ray of the maternal abdomen generally suggests a gestational age of at least 36 weeks and the upper tibial epiphysis that the duration of pregnancy is between 38 and 42 weeks. However, the appearance of these epiphyses is delayed when there is intrauterine growth retardation.

3. Hydramnios (an abbreviation of polyhydramnios) is the term used when there is a clinical impression or ultrasound evidence of excess amniotic fluid. Fetal parts are usually difficult to palpate and the uterus often appears tense and large for dates. A fluid thrill can usually be elicited. The amniotic fluid volume usually exceeds 1.5 l when hydramnios is clinically evident. A semiquantitative assessment can be made using ultrasound. The possibility of undiagnosed multiple pregnancy must always be considered when excess amniotic fluid is detected. The condition is also more common in women with carbohydrate intolerance. A glucose tolerance test should therefore be performed to exclude gestational diabetes. Several congenital anomalies are associated with polyhdramnios. These include neural tube defects (e.g. anencephaly and spina bifida) and gastrointestinal abnormalities (e.g. oesophageal and duodenal atresia and tracheo-oesophageal fistula). Careful ultrasound examination should therefore always be performed to exclude an abnormality of the fetal spine or head. (Abdominal X-rays may be misleading and are now seldom used to assess fetal bony abnormalities.) Other rarer causes of polyhydramnios include rhesus and non-rhesus hydrops, placental chorioangiomas, fetal retroperitoneal fibrosis, and renal anomalies associated with fetal polyuria.

If it is necessary to rupture the membranes of a woman with polyhydramnios, care should be taken to prevent rapid escape of the amniotic fluid as this may cause a placental abruption.

A stomach tube should always be passed on the baby immediately after delivery to exclude fetal oesophageal atresia.

A 42-year-old lecturer's wife attended the antenatal clinic to book for hospital confinement at 14 weeks in her fifth pregnancy. She had three children aged 19, 14 and 6 years. All had been delivered normally at term. Her third pregnancy had ended as a spontaneous abortion 7 years earlier at 8 weeks.

After 7 weeks of amenorrhoea in the current pregnancy, she had experienced severe palpitations, become very tired and suffered marked weight loss. Investigation had shown her to be thyrotoxic and treatment with carbimazole 10 mg t.i.d. had been started at 10 weeks gestation. Her past medical history included an appendicectomy at the age of 13 years, excision of a cold thyroid nodule at the age of 31 and pleurisy in her fourth pregnancy. Several of her relatives had died of cardiovascular disease and an uncle and an aunt had developed maturity onset diabetes. She was allergic to Elastoplast and penicillin.

On examination she was underweight (50.4 kg) for her height (160 cm) and had moderate exophthalmos. Thyroid examination revealed an overlying scar and slight diffuse enlargement of the gland. Her breasts were tense but otherwise normal. Abdominal examination demonstrated a 14-week uterus and an appendicectomy scar. Bimanual pelvic examination confirmed the uterine size and was otherwise normal.

All the routine antenatal booking investigations were normal. Arrangements were made to perform an amniocentesis at 16 weeks to karyotype the fetus and measure the amniotic fluid alpha-fetoprotein concentration.

1. How would you assess thyroid function in a pregnant patient?
2. How would you manage this patient's pregnancy and puerperium?
3. What is the risk of Down's syndrome in this patient?

1. The high metabolic activity of the fetoplacental unit causes an increase in basal metabolic rate during pregnancy. This is associated with a number of physiological changes which may mimic mild hyperthyroidism, including heat intolerance, increased sweating and a raised pulse rate. In addition, slight diffuse thyroid enlargement usually occurs during normal pregnancy. However, as these changes do not indicate a true functional alteration of thyroid function during pregnancy, clinical assessment of thyroid function in the pregnant woman is difficult. Biochemically, an oestrogen-induced increase in the production of thyroid binding globulin (TBG) by the liver results in a significant increase in the serum protein-bound iodine concentration. There is, however, no significant increase in the free thyroxine concentration which is the critical factor in the control of metabolism by the thyroid gland.

    Thyroid function is, therefore, most simply assessed during pregnancy by measuring the true free thyroxine (FT_4) concentration. Alternatively, the free thyroxine index (FT_4I) can be measured. This involves measuring the total thyroxine (T_4) and relating it to the amount of protein available for binding with T_4. This relationship remains unaltered during pregnancy because both the amount of T_4 and protein available to bind it increase in similar proportions. Some laboratories measure T_4 binding globulin directly, but in most an estimate is obtained by measuring the red cell or resin triiodothyronine (T_3) uptake when radioactive T_3 mixed with serum is added. In pregnancy the higher thyroglobulin levels cause more radioactive T_3 to become protein bound leaving less radioactive T_3 to be taken up by the red cells or resin. The values for the T_3 resin uptake test are therefore lower in pregnant than in non-pregnant women. The product of total T_4 concentration (elevated by the increase in TBG) and the T_3 resin uptake (reduced by T_3 binding to the increased TBG) divided by 100 gives the free thyroxine index, $FT_4I = T_4$ (ug/dl) x T_3 uptake (%) / 100, which in normal pregnancy falls in the same range as in the non-pregnant patient.

    Radioactive ^{123}I uptake scans are contraindicated in pregnancy as the radioactive iodine crosses the placenta and is concentrated in the fetal thyroid, causing neonatal hypothyroidism and cretinism.

2. Hyperthyroidism is 3–5 times more common in women than men. Although untreated thyrotoxicosis is associated with reduced fertility, it occurs in approximately 1 in 1500 pregnancies. The condition is generally well tolerated by the mother, but there is an increased incidence of abortion, premature labour, pre-eclampsia and postpartum haemorrhage. The treatment of thyrotoxicosis during pregnancy involves control of the signs and symptoms of the disease with carbimazole or propylthiouracil, both of which cross the placenta. Large doses of these drugs (carbimazole 50–100 mg daily; propylthiouracil 100–150 mg 6-hourly) are given initially until symptoms abate. The dose should then be reduced to the lowest possible level consistent with the maintenance of euthyroid state, until delivery. Serial measurement of the FT_4 or FT_4I are the single most useful tests for following the response to therapy; however the fetal heart rate is also a good index of maternal thyroid status, being commonly above 160 beats/minute

in uncontrolled thyrotoxicosis and less than 110 beats/minute in myxoedema. Hypothyroidism should be avoided, but concomitant administration of thyroxine or tri-iodothyronine is not necessary. If the mother is maintained meticulously in the euthyroid state the fetus does not appear to be a risk, but if the mother is hypothyroid then fetus is also likely to be. If treatment is started early, as in this patient, it can frequently be stopped a week or two before delivery. If the disease is well controlled, no special precautions need be taken during labour. If the mother remains on antithyroid drugs during the puerperium, then breast feeding is contraindicated as these compounds are secreted in breast milk. The incidence of neonatal thyrotoxicosis is about 2%. This is a serious problem and the baby should always be examined carefully by a paediatrician.

Surgical treatment is rarely advocated and, for the reasons already mentioned, radioactive iodine should never be given during pregnancy for diagnosis or treatment.

3. The risk of Down's syndrome is approximately 1:2000 at 25; 1:350 at 35; 1:200 at 37; 1:100 at 40; 1:70 at 42 and 1:40 at 44 years of age.

Obstetrics 26

A 31-year-old primigravid Australian teacher, married to a research assistant, booked for antenatal care after 16 weeks of amenorrhoea. Her menstrual cycle had been regular with periods every 28 days and she had not used any contraception for 2 years. She was a fit woman who had no relevant past medical history. Her mother was hypertensive, her grandmother diabetic and she had a twin sister. She had used oral contraception during the first 7 years of her marriage and the sheath for 2 years after this. She conceived a year after they had stopped using contraception. She smoked 15 cigarettes a day before the pregnancy but had reduced to 5 a day shortly after missing her period.

On examination she was a tall (170 cm) fit-looking woman, who was not obese (65.2 kg). Her blood pressure was 140/80 mmHg and there was no abnormality on general examination. Her breasts were normal. Abdominal palpation revealed a 16-week size uterus. Her vulva, vagina and cervix were normal. Bimanual palpation confirmed the uterine size and there were no adnexal masses.

All booking investigations, including a serum alpha-fetoprotein estimation, were normal.

Her pregnancy progressed normally and subsequent blood pressure recordings were in the range 120–130/70–80 mmHg. The fetal lie was transverse at 32 weeks, but cephalic thereafter. At 38 weeks a moderate degree of hydramnios was noted. The fetal and uterine size were compatible with her dates, but the fetal head was high and free. It did, however engage when she was standing. An ultrasound scan was performed to exclude placenta praevia and estimate fetal size. The placenta was situated in the upper segment, mainly on the posterior wall. The BPD measured 9.6 cm, the head circumference 33 cm and the abdominal circumference 34.5 cm. The amniotic fluid volume was reported to be slightly increased. She was seen weekly thereafter until 41 weeks and, although the head remained high when she was supine, there was no other abnormality. The day after her last antenatal visit she came to the labour ward, in a state of panic, as she had not felt any fetal movements at all for about 16 hours. On examination her uterus was soft and non-tender. The fetal lie remained longitudinal with a cephalic presentation. Careful auscultation with a Pinard stethoscope failed to detect the fetal heart and a diagnosis of intrauterine death was made.

1. What investigations would you perform to confirm this diagnosis?
2. How would you manage this patient?

1. Real time ultrasound examination of the fetal heart provides the definitive diagnosis of intrauterine death. If this equipment is not available, then the fetal heart tones can be sought with a Doppler ultrasound device. The fetal X-ray changes, which used to be the only way of confirming fetal death, take several days to develop and are seldom used nowadays, except in centres without an ultrasound scanner. The three most important radiological signs of fetal death are overlap of the skull bones (Spalding's sign); gas in the heart and major blood vessels (Robert's sign) and an abnormal fetal posture with exaggeration of spinal curvature. Spalding's sign is not reliable if the patient is in labour, or has ruptured membranes, as moulding of the head of a live fetus produces a similar X-ray appearance. Application of an electrode to the fetus in an attempt to record the fetal heart rate should not be used to diagnose fetal death. This is because the automatic gain used in fetal heart rate monitors means that even a small maternal heart ECG signal will be detected and will result in a heart rate recording which may be misinterpreted as that from the fetus, particularly if the mother has a tachycardia.

2. Seventy five per cent of patients with intrauterine fetal death will go into labour within 14 days and 90% within 21 days. Because it may be difficult to induce labour, especially if the cervix is unfavourable, some obstetricians prefer to await such spontaneous onset. Many women, however, find the waiting involved emotionally difficult to accept. Another disadvantage of waiting is that disseminated intravascular coagulation may develop if thromboplastins from the dead fetus and placenta enter the maternal circulation. This risk increases with the passage of time, reaching 25% at 5 weeks. A plasma fibrinogen estimation should, therefore, always be made when intrauterine death is diagnosed. If hypofibrinogenaemia is detected, intravenous heparin therapy should be given while labour is induced, provided there is no evidence of bleeding.

   Labour should be induced using intravaginal prostaglandin E_2 (5 mg in tablet, gel or pessary form). If labour is not established within 6 hours, a further dose of prostaglandin should be given. If labour has still not begun after 12 hours intravenous oxytocin should be given. This infusion should commence at 2 mu per minute and increase to a maximum of 32 mu per minute. Because of the antidiuretic effect of this hormone, the infusion should ideally be administered using a syringe pump to minimise the amount of fluid administered. A careful fluid balance chart should be maintained to ensure that water intoxication is avoided. If labour is not established after 12–16 hours of oxytocin administration, it is preferable to stop the infusion, repeat the prostaglandin treatment and, after the patient has had a night's rest, recommence oxytocin therapy. Alternatively, extra-amniotic infusion of prostaglandin at a rate of 1 mg per hour via a Foley catheter can be used. Amniotomy is contraindicated when the fetus is dead because of the risk of introducing bacteria into the uterine cavity, whose contents form a near perfect culture medium.

Throughout this difficult time the parents must be treated with compassion. Adequate pain relief should be provided in labour, but heavy sedation should be avoided. Epidural anaesthesia is ideal provided there is no evidence of coagulopathy. Both parents should be told that grief is a normal reaction. They should be encouraged, but not forced, to see and hold the baby, even if it is macerated or deformed. Maternal fantasies of the dead newborn are often far worse than reality. Photographs should always be taken in case the parents initially refuse to see the baby, but later wish they had. Mementoes such as locks of the baby's hair can also be kept. Lactation should be suppressed using oral bromocriptine if necessary. Gentle but firm requests must be made for permission to perform an autopsy and take whole body X-rays. Whenever possible, fetal blood should also be obtained for karyotyping to exclude a chromosomal abnormality or unsuspected haemolytic disease.

A maternal blood sample should be taken for glycosylated haemoglobin (HbA$_1$c) estimation to exclude gestational diabetes.

Subsequent pregnancies should be treated as high risk, the patient seen more frequently and monitored fully. Such monitoring has no proven medical benefit, but is emotionally valuable to both mother and obstetrician, and harmless so long as premature intervention is not undertaken for minor deviations from normality. If the intrauterine death occurred late in pregnancy, elective induction of the subsequent labour before the critical date can also be reassuring for the mother and carries little risk, providing it is at 38 weeks gestation or later. A glucose tolerance test (GTT) should be performed at 28 weeks in the next pregnancy, as it is more reliable at indicating minor degrees of carbohydrate intolerance than a postpartum test.

This patient's stillborn baby weighed 3.68 kg and no fetal abnormality was detected on postmortem examination. There was, however, a true knot in the umbilical cord, which may have been the cause of death.

Obstetrics 27

A 22-year-old married hairdresser attended the antenatal booking clinic after 16 weeks amenorrhoea in her second pregnancy. She had been epileptic since the age of 13 years and was taking phenytoin 300 mg daily. She had not had a fit for 6 years. Her first pregnancy 2 years earlier had been normal, but her son had been delivered with forceps because of poor maternal effort in the second stage of labour. There was no other relevant past medical or family history. She had used a combined oral contraceptive pill for 2 years before her first pregnancy and an intrauterine contraceptive device (IUCD) for a year after the birth. Her menstrual cycle had been very irregular since removal of the IUCD with scanty bleeds of 1–4 days duration at intervals of between 4 and 12 weeks.

Despite this, the uterine size on abdominal and pelvic examination was compatible with 16 weeks gestation and this was confirmed by an ultrasound measurement of the fetal biparietal diameter. She was noted to be overweight (67 kg) for her height (158 cm), but there was no other abnormality on general or pelvic examination. Her blood pressure was 130/80 mmHg.

Her pregnancy progressed normally until 32 weeks when her blood pressure was found to be 150/100 mmHg.

She was noted to have gained an excessive amount of weight (12 kg) in the previous 16 weeks and complained that she became tired quickly. Abdominal examination revealed that the uterine and fetal size corresponded with her dates. The lie was longitudinal and the presentation cephalic. Her abdominal striae were noted to be unusually wide and deep purple in colour. Similar striae were present on both thighs. Her obesity was mainly of the face and trunk and she had quite severe acne. There was no oedema. Urine analysis revealed glucose + on dipstick testing, but there was no proteinuria.

1. What is the likely diagnosis in this case?
2. How would you manage the remainder of the pregnancy?
3. What is the effect of pregnancy on epilepsy?
4. What effect does maternal anticonvulsant therapy have on the fetus?

1. This patient displayed many of the features of Cushing's syndrome, namely oligomenorrhoea, truncal and facial obesity, acne, exaggerated purple striae on her abdomen and thighs, fatigue, hypertension and glycosuria.

    Cushing's syndrome is usually associated with secondary amenorrhoea and it is exceedingly rare for women with this condition to become pregnant. This patient had experienced oligomenorrhoea for a year and, presumably, if she had not become pregnant would ultimately have developed amenorrhoea due to the disease.

    Pregnancy is associated with an increase in both bound and free circulating cortisol. The increase in bound cortisol results largely from an increased hepatic production of cortisol-binding globulin induced by placental oestrogens. In late pregnancy plasma bound cortisol concentrations are on average 2–3 times higher than those of non-pregnant women and there is a parallel increase in unbound cortisol concentrations to levels which may overlap those seen in Cushing's syndrome. Because pregnancy mimics many of the features of the syndrome it is easily overlooked clinically and can be difficult to diagnose biochemically. Day–night variation of plasma unbound cortisol, which is lost in Cushing's syndrome, however, persists in pregnancy, albeit at a reduced level. The diagnosis was confirmed in this case by measurement of 9 a.m. and midnight plasma unbound cortisol concentrations, which were virtually identical and well above the normal range for late pregnancy. Ultrasound scanning subsequently demonstrated a right adrenal tumour. Glucose tolerance is frequently impaired in this condition, but despite her glycosuria, this patient had a normal glucose tolerance test. Her electrolyte concentrations were also normal, but the serum potassium was low and only just within the normal range.

2. Cushing's syndrome occurs three times more commonly in women than in men and, despite its rarity, should always be borne in mind when unexplained hypertension occurs in pregnancy. Fifty to 70% of cases are due to an adrenal adenoma, 20–30% an adrenal carcinoma and 10–20% have a pituitary adenoma. The incidence of ectopic tumours has not been fully evaluated. The outcome of pregnancy in this condition is poor and in 26 cases reported between 1952 and 1972 the incidence of abortion was 20%, premature labour 8% and stillbirth 10%. If the diagnosis is made early in pregnancy, and a tumour can be identified, surgical treatment is advocated. If the diagnosis is made late in pregnancy careful fetal monitoring should be performed and delivery effected at 37–38 weeks, both to reduce the chance of late stillbirth and to reduce the risk of spinal collapse secondary to osteoporosis. Although there is no contraindication to vaginal delivery, this patient was delivered by caesarean section because of a breech presentation and an apparently large baby. Neonatal adrenal insufficiency has been reported in association with maternal Cushing's syndrome and the newborn should therefore be carefully monitored in a special care unit for the first 48–72 hours after delivery.

    Detailed investigation of this patient, commenced 2 weeks after delivery, and including both a CAT scan and arteriogram, confirmed the right adrenal mass, and endocrine investigation, including failure of dexamethasone suppression, confirmed excessive autonomous adrenal cortisol production. Histological examination of the right adrenal removed a month after delivery confirmed a benign adenoma.

3. Provided adequate anticonvulsant therapy is maintained, pregnancy does not appear to have an adverse effect on epilepsy. Three factors may affect serum concentrations of anticonvulsants during pregnancy, namely increased protein binding, increased volume of distribution (due to the 45% increase in plasma volume), and changes in gastrointestinal absorption. During pregnancy, serum anticonvulsant levels should therefore be monitored regularly and the dose adjusted to maintain concentrations in the therapeutic range. Folic acid supplements should also be given as most major anticonvulsants (including phenytoin) may induce folate deficiency.

4. There is an increase in the incidence of congenital malformation (especially cleft palate and cardiac disease) in infants born to epileptics. Although phenytoin has been the most frequently implicated drug, it is also the most widely used. Valproic acid has been recommended in preference, but congenital malformations, particularly spina bifida, have also occurred when women have taken this newer drug. It is unclear, at present, whether the increased risk of malformation results from a common genetic predisposition in epileptics, deficiency states induced by drugs, or a direct drug effect. At present there is insufficient evidence to justify changing drug therapy prior to planned conception or during early pregnancy.

Obstetrics 28

The patient, a 24-year-old shop assistant, had been married for 6 years to a welder. Their first child had been delivered 4 years earlier in a cottage hospital. The pregnancy and labour had been entirely normal. She attended the antenatal booking clinic at 16 weeks gestation in her second pregnancy. Her dates were certain and the pregnancy had been progressing normally. She had never had a blood transfusion and there was no relevant past medical or family history. General examination was normal and abdominal palpation revealed that the uterine size was compatible with her dates. An ultrasound scan confirmed the duration of pregnancy and the routine booking investigations were normal, apart from the antibody screen. This showed the presence of anti-D antibodies in a concentration of 0.47 iu ml (0.09 μg/ml). Her blood group was A rhesus negative and that of her husband A rhesus positive with a genotype of CDe/CDe. Repeat measurements of her antibody concentrations at 20, 24 and 28 weeks gestation were 0.66, 2.2 and 24 iu/ml. Apart from these findings the pregnancy appeared to be progressing normally.

1. Why do you think this patient has developed rhesus antibodies?
2. What is the significance of these results?
3. What further investigation would you perform?
4. What treatment would you give?
5. What is the significance of her husband's genotype?

1. Rhesus isoimmunisation occurs when fetal cells of a rhesus positive fetus enter the circulation of a rhesus negative mother. This usually occurs at the time of delivery or abortion. If the fetal cells are ABO incompatible with the mother (e.g. the baby is A and the mother is B), they are destroyed by antibodies circulating in the mother's blood. If however they are ABO compatible (e.g. the same blood group, or the mother is AB, universal recipient) then the fetal cells persist in the mother's circulation. After a few days the mother's immune system begins to react against the unfamiliar rhesus antigen. Initially IgM antibodies are produced which do not cross the placenta, but later IgG antibodies, which do cross the placenta, are produced. These antibodies are usually formed against the D antigen and are hence called anti-D antibodies. (Anti-C and anti-E antibodies may also form if the mother lacks these antigens and they are present on the fetal red cells.) Sensitisation may also occur following amniocentesis, antepartum haemorrhage (APH) and external cephalic version (ECV).

2. As these latter events did not occur in this patient's first or current pregnancy it seems likely that prophylactic anti-D administration was either overlooked in her first pregnancy, or an inadequate amount of antibody was administered. It is usual to give 500 IU units of anti-D antibody within 60 hours of delivery to all rhesus negative women who deliver a rhesus positive baby. This is, however, only sufficient to eliminate 4 ml of rhesus D positive blood from the maternal circulation. The size of the fetomaternal bleed should, therefore, always be assessed by determining the quantity of fetal cells in maternal blood using the Kleihauer test. If the estimated volume exceeds 4 ml then the amount of anti-D given should be increased accordingly. 250 IU of anti-D immunoglobulin is usually administered to the mother immediately after abortion, amniocentesis, ECV or minor APH.

3. A quantitative assay for maternal plasma anti-D concentrations is now available. This has enabled a much more precise estimation of anti-D levels to be achieved than was possible using anti-D titres. Significant fetal haemolysis is likely with values in excess of 2.5 iu/ml. At one time, in order to assess the degree to which the fetus was being affected, it was necessary to perform an amniocentesis. This allowed the measurement of the bilirubin content of the amniotic fluid, which reflected the rate of fetal haemolysis. The measurement was made by optical density analysis, and the degree of haemolysis estimated by plotting on a Liley chart. Nowadays, all this can be side-stepped by direct measurement of the fetal haemoglobin concentration obtained by cordocentesis. The rapid rise in anti-D concentration in this patient suggested a major fetomaternal bleed. In response to the high anti-D concentration at 28 weeks, cordocentesis was performed. Fetal haemoglobin concentration was only 6 g/dl and an intrauterine transfusion was performed. The donor rhesus positive blood was injected directly into the umbilical vein. Repeat transfusions were necessary at 30, 32 and 34 weeks gestation. Since the fetal loss rate is approximately 0.5–1% at each

cordocentesis, it is usually preferable to deliver after 34 weeks rather than risk further transfusions. In this case, labour was induced at 35 weeks with intravaginal prostaglandin E_2 gel. A 2.1 kg male infant in good condition was born spontaneously after a 9-hour labour. He required only one exchange transfusion and subsequently did well.

4. Rhesus disease is now rare in developed countries and management of affected pregnancies should be confined to centres where the expertise for cordocentesis is readily available. Although all now use the technique to assess the need for, and amount of, intrauterine transfusion, some prefer to use the older technique of intraperitoneal transfusion for giving the blood. They claim it reduces the risk of sudden fetal circulatory overload, and is associated with a lower fetal mortality.

5. Her husband is homozygous for the rhesus D antigen. All their subsequent children will be rhesus positive.

Obstetrics 29

A 34-year-old Negro woman was referred by her family doctor for an urgent consultant antenatal opinion because of slight suprapubic pain and vaginal bleeding at 17 weeks gestation. She had been trying to have a child for nearly 10 years. A laparoscopy 4 years earlier had shown normal ovaries and patent tubes. There were, however, some peritubal adhesions and a small pedunculated fundal fibroid. To her great delight, she conceived a year later without treatment, but unfortunately miscarried at 10 weeks. An evacuation of retained products of conception was performed at this time. The following year she again conceived. This sadly proved to be a tubal ectopic pregnancy and a left salpingectomy was performed after 8 weeks amenorrhoea. The present pregnancy, her third, was confirmed by an ultrasound scan at 11 weeks. Her booking investigations, including a sickle cell test, were normal, apart from her haemoglobin which was only 7.8 g/dl. The haematological indices and blood film suggested iron deficiency. Red cell fragility studies and a haemoglobin electrophoresis were normal. She was therefore admitted, given a transfusion of 4 units of packed cells and started on oral iron and folic acid. At 16 weeks the uterine size was compatible with 18 weeks gestation. Because she complained of some lower abdominal discomfort and was naturally anxious about the pregnancy, the fetal heart was demonstrated to her using Doppler ultrasound. It was also planned to perform a repeat ultrasound scan at her next antenatal visit. To everyone's surprise, her haemoglobin at this visit was still only 8.4 g/dl and she was therefore given a further 3-unit blood transfusion. There was no history of bleeding and neither her urine nor stools contained occult blood. Ten days later she was admitted complaining that she had experienced gradually increasing lower abdominal discomfort over the preceding week. On the morning of admission she had experienced severe backache. She had also lost some 'tissue' mixed with blood and had subsequently noticed a blood-stained vaginal discharge. She had no other complaints nor any relevant past medical history. She was not taking any medication other than oral iron and folic acid supplements.

On examination she looked fit. Her temperature was 36.9°C, her blood pressure was 110/60 mmHg and her pulse rate 88 beats per minute. Abdominal palpation revealed a mass arising centrally from the pelvis, which was compatible with a uterus of 22 weeks gestation. This was not tender, but there was some discomfort on palpation in the right iliac fossa. Pelvic examination confirmed the abdominal findings. There did not appear to be any other pelvic mass. Her cervix was closed and there was a slight brownish vaginal discharge. To the dismay of all concerned, careful examination with Doppler ultrasound failed to detect the fetal heart. Her haemoglobin at this time was 10.2 g/dl.

1. What is the differential diagnosis?
2. Can you explain her recurrent anaemia?
3. What investigations would you perform?

1. This patient presented an extremely difficult clinical problem, one that caused considerable confusion, and concern, to those responsible for her care.

   At first sight the diagnosis appeared to be a missed abortion. Although the uterine size is usually smaller than expected with this condition, a lethal congenital abnormality associated with polyhydramnios could explain why this patient's uterus appeared larger than her dates. Intrauterine death associated with placental separation and a large retroplacental bleed would also cause the uterus to be enlarged. The lack of uterine tenderness, does, however, make this diagnosis rather unlikely, even though abruption of a placenta situated on the posterior uterine wall may only cause slight uterine tenderness and backache. This diagnosis would, however, explain the history of vaginal bleeding and slight anaemia at the time of her admission.

   A hydatidiform mole is another possibility. It is, however, rare for this condition to occur in association with a normal intrauterine pregnancy. It would, on the other hand, explain the enlarged uterus, loss of 'tissue' and vaginal bleeding observed in this case.

   Enlargement of the fundal fibroid, noted during laparoscopy 4 years earlier, could also explain why the uterus appeared large for dates. Red degeneration of this fibroid is also a remote possibility. This process, however, usually produces a pyrexia and severe abdominal pain; it seldom causes fetal demise. Furthermore, in common with all the other diagnoses listed above, it fails to explain two episodes of severe anaemia, earlier in the pregnancy, which had necessitated transfusion of 7 units of blood.

2. When a patient who is known to have had a previous ectopic pregnancy presents with this history and the above findings on clinical examination,the possibility of an extrauterine pregnancy must be considered. The ultrasound report at 11 weeks may appear to exclude this, but when the fetus is growing normally an early ultrasound scan may easily mistake an extrauterine pregnancy for one which is intrauterine. This diagnosis would also explain her recurrent anaemia. As the extrauterine placenta grows it invades adjacent pelvic and abdominal blood vessels and intermittent bleeding occurs. This is contained by surrounding omentum and bowel and may produce only minimal discomfort. The gestation sac surrounded by organising clot may mimic a uterus which is enlarging normally. The fetus may survive for many weeks in the midst of this anatomical chaos, but usually develops compression defects and ultimately succumbs from placental insufficiency.

3. A careful ultrasound scan should always be performed when the condition is suspected and, as in this case, may prove to be diagnostic. The scan was reported as showing, 'A bulky uterus with no evidence of an intrauterine pregnancy. Most of the abdominal mass consists of solid and transonic areas and appears to be blood clot. A fetus is present on the left side of the mass. Its head is flattened. No fetal heart movements can be seen. Conclusion — an extrauterine pregnancy surrounded by a large organising blood clot'.

On examination under anaesthesia the uterus could be palpated separate from the mass and the uterine cavity was only 9 cm in length. Laparotomy confirmed the ultrasound findings. The placenta had implanted onto the right ovarian vessels, broad ligament, omentum and some small bowel. It is usually best not to attempt removal of the placenta in advanced abdominal pregnancies because of the catastrophic haemorrhage that this may produce. In this case, as in most extrauterine pregnancies that are diagnosed early, it was,however, possible to remove the entire pregnancy.

With hindsight, the 'tissue' that this patient passed on the day of her admission to hospital was probably decidua.

Obstetrics 30

A 22-year-old primigravid kitchen assistant, who was married to a roof-felt fixer, first attended the antenatal clinic at 17 weeks. She had a regular 28 days menstrual cycle and was certain of the date of her last period. She was noted to be of short stature (146 cm), but was not overweight (47 kg). She gave a history of postcoital cystitis since the onset of sexual activity, but a midstream urine (MSU) specimen obtained at the booking visit showed no growth on culture. On examination her uterus appeared slightly large for dates (approximately 20 weeks size). This was thought to be due to her height, as an ultrasound biparietal diameter measurement a week later confirmed her dates and excluded multiple pregnancy.

The pregnancy remained entirely normal until 31 weeks, when she was admitted complaining of frequency and dysuria for a week. After the symptoms had been present for 4 days, she consulted her general practitioner who had prescribed cotrimoxazole, but as this had made her feel unwell she had stopped taking it after only 48 hours. During the following 24 hours she had felt feverish and had developed generalised backache and intermittent lower abdominal pain. She had lost her appetite, felt nauseous and had vomited several times. There was no other relevant past medical or family history.

On examination she was flushed and looked unwell. Her temperature was 38.6°C, pulse rate 100 beats/minute and blood pressure 110/70 mm Hg. She appeared to be slightly dehydrated, but despite this had mild ankle oedema. There was no abnormality on examination of her respiratory or cardiovascular systems. Abdominal palpation revealed uterine enlargement with a symphysis–fundal height of 34 cm. The uterus was tense but there was no uterine tenderness. The fetus was difficult to palpate, but the lie appeared to be longitudinal with an engaged cephalic presentation. The fetal heart was heard and the rate was about 170 beats/minute. Abdominal palpation revealed slight suprapubic tenderness, marked bilateral loin tenderness and slight guarding, but no rebound tenderness. Vaginal examination confirmed that the presentation was cephalic. The cervix was 2 cm dilated and 1–2 cm long and the membranes were noted to be 'bulging'. There was no sign of bleeding.

1. Make a diagnosis and describe the aetiology of this condition.
2. What investigations would you perform and how would you treat this patient?
3. What further information do you require about this patient?
4. Comment on the treatment prescribed by her family doctor.

1. This patient has acute pyelonephritis. She gave a history of recurrent urinary tract infection, and, although asymptomatic bacteriuria is common in pregnancy (2–10% depending on the population studied), the screening MSU obtained at her first antenatal visit was sterile. She therefore appears to have acquired cystitis de novo during the second trimester, presumably as an ascending infection, and probably following coitus.

   Dilatation of the upper urinary tract occurs in most pregnancies. It can be demonstrated on the right side in 90% of women and on the left side in 60% and appears to be due both to relaxation of ureteric smooth muscle (caused by progesterone) and compression of the ureters (especially the right) by the enlarging uterus and dilated ovarian vessels. These changes predispose to ascending bacterial infection and pyelonephritis, usually due to *Escherischia coli* or less commonly *Proteus* or *Klebsiella* species. Urgent microscopy of an MSU obtained from this patient showed 1000 pus cells/mm^3 and the urine contained 1 g of protein/litre. Her blood urea and electrolyte results were normal. Intravenous fluids and amoxycillin 500 mg and metronidazole 500 mg 8-hourly by intravenous injection were commenced. Subsequent urine culture confirmed *E. coli* as the causative organism. Blood culture was negative.

2. Acute pyelonephritis is frequently associated with premature labour and the history and findings in this patient suggest that her uterus may be contracting. The fetal heart rate of 170 beats/minute may be secondary to the maternal pyrexia, but could also be due to fetal hypoxia. A continuous cardiotocograph recording was therefore obtained. Although this showed that she was not contracting, it confirmed a baseline fetal heart rate of 160–170 beats/minute with marked loss of baseline variability and successive prolonged decelerations which were unrelated to the patient's posture. These occurred approximately every 10 minutes, lasted for between 4 and 9 minutes and the fetal heart rate dropped to 70 beats/minute with each deceleration. As it was impossible to exclude a concealed placental abruption or intrauterine infection secondary to maternal septicaemia, it was decided to deliver the baby by emergency caesarean section. At operation the liquor appeared infected and there was no evidence of abruptio placentae. The baby, a boy who weighed 1.82 kg, was extremely ill. His Apgar scores were 1 at 5 minutes, 2 at 10 minutes and 6 at 15 minutes. The cord vein pH at delivery was 7.14. The baby was treated with penicillin and gentamicin but died 24 hours after delivery.

3. This case highlights the extremely serious sequelae of pyelonephritis during pregnancy. As 30% of women with asymptomatic bacteria will develop pyelonephritis, this condition should always be excluded in early pregnancy. Patients with a history of recurrent urinary tract infection before pregnancy should have serial MSU specimens sent for culture during pregnancy. Finally, when asymptomatic bacteriuria is detected in pregnancy, or a symptomatic infection occurs, the importance of completing any course of therapy that is prescribed must be impressed upon

the patient. An MSU specimen should be sent for culture at every subsequent antenatal visit after completion of therapy to exclude recurrent infection.

4. Cotrimoxazole contains folic acid antagonists and, although it has been widely used in late pregnancy without apparent harm, is considered (by the manufacturers) to be contraindicated because of a theoretical risk to the fetus. This drug combination (trimethoprim and sulphamethoxazole) is therefore best avoided in pregnancy. If there is no other suitable antimicrobial agent, then a folic acid supplement (5–10 mg daily) should be given in addition to the cotrimoxazole. It should never be given to the patients with impaired folate status, e.g. epileptics.

Obstetrics 31

A 23-year-old nurse booked at 15 weeks in her first pregnancy. She had stopped using oral contraception 3 years earlier, had a regular 30–32 day menstrual cycle, was certain of the date of her last period and had a positive pregnancy test after 6 weeks amenorrhoea. There was no relevant past medical or family history.

Examination at this time revealed her to be a fit, healthy young woman of short stature (140 cm), but normal weight for her height (42.8 kg). Her husband, who was also a nurse, was noted to be 183 cm tall. She was booked for hospital confinement, but antenatal care was shared with her general practitioner. The pregnancy progressed normally, but at 38 weeks the fetal head was four-fifths palpable above the pelvic inlet on abdominal examination. The uterine and fetal size were compatible with her dates. The fetal head did not engage in the pelvis with sitting or standing.

1. List the possible causes of a high head at 38 weeks gestation.
2. How would you manage this patient?
3. What is the effect of paternal stature on fetal size?

1. The most likely cause of a high head in a patient of this stature is cephalopelvic disproportion. Other possibilities must, however, be borne in mind and excluded. The most important of these is placenta praevia. Although this condition usually causes some vaginal bleeding before 38 weeks of pregnancy, haemorrhage may occur only when labour starts. Multiple pregnancy seems unlikely, but the possibility of a head (or breech) deeply engaged in the pelvis and another head free above the pelvic inlet must be considered. One of the commoner causes is a deflexed head in the occipitoposterior position. Further extension to produce a face or brow presentation increases the presenting diameter and impairs descent of the head into the pelvis. In a woman with a pelvis of normal size cephalopelvic disproportion may be due to hydrocephalus or a very large baby. Polyhydramnios is also frequently associated with a high head. Although rare, a pelvic tumour such as an ovarian cyst or cervical or lower segment fibroid will prevent engagement of the head. An even rarer cause of a high head is advanced extrauterine (intra-abdominal) pregnancy, although this is often associated with an oblique lie. In practice, a full bladder or rectum is probably the commonest cause of all. Finally it should be remembered that in some ethnic groups, such as the West African, engagement of the fetal head often does not occur until the onset of labour, probably because of the high inclination of the pelvic inlet in these women, combined with minor degrees of CPD.

2. In the first instance an ultrasound scan should be performed to localise the placenta and exclude an undiagnosed twin, hydrocephalus or a pelvic tumour. Having excluded a placenta praevia, a thorough pelvic examination should be performed to assess the pelvic shape and dimensions and exclude a bony abnormality of the pelvis. If there is no suggestion of absolute cephalopelvic disproportion (i.e. an anteroposterior pelvic inlet diameter of less than 10.0 cm) or an exceptionally large baby, then it is reasonable to allow a trial of labour. If there is doubt, an erect lateral pelvimetry should be performed, although this will be unnecessary in most cases.

    A scan in this patient demonstrated a fundal placenta and pelvic examination confirmed a symmetrically small pelvis of normal shape with an estimated true conjugate diameter of 9.6 cm. This was confirmed on X-ray and, because the baby appeared relatively large (3.4 kg), she was delivered by elective lower segment caesarean section.

3. Paternal stature has a very limited impact on the fetal size. In statistical terms, less than 10% of the variation in birthweight can be explained by the height of the father, and in clinical practice it can be ignored. Maternal height does, however, have an important influence on fetal size, although, as this case demonstrates, the constraint which short stature imposes on fetal growth does not ensure that the fetal size is appropriate for the maternal pelvic size. In statistical terms, variation in maternal height only explains about 20% of the variation in birthweight; maternal weight for height is a more important determinant of fetal size. A maternal body mass index (BMI: weight in kg divided by height in metres

squared, kg/m^2) of >30 trebles the chance of birthweight exceeding the 90th centile, weight for gestational age, whereas a BMI of <19 trebles the chance of birthweight being less than the 10th centile.

Obstetrics 32

A 21-year-old typist, who was married to an electrician, attended the antenatal booking clinic after 12 weeks amenorrhoea. Her menstrual cycle had previously been regular with 6 days bleeding every 28 days.

A pregnancy test performed by her general practitioner was positive. She had stopped oral contraception a year earlier and this was her first pregnancy. There was no significant past medical or family history. Her weight was 48.8 kg and her height 157 cm.

There was no abnormality on general examination. Her breasts were normal. The uterine fundus was just palpable at the level of the pubic symphysis. Vaginal examination revealed a complete longitudinal vaginal septum and a double cervix. The septum was soft and easily distensible, it separated the two cervices completely at the upper end of the vagina and extended down to the level of the hymen. The left cervix appeared to be larger than that on the right side. Bimanual examination showed the uterus to be the correct size for 12 weeks gestation. It appeared to be symmetrical in outline. There were no adnexal masses.

1. What is the cause of this abnormality?
2. What other congenital anomalies may be associated with this abnormality?
3. How would you manage this pregnancy?
4. What obstetric complications would you anticipate?

1. The vagina above the hymen appears to develop from a
    proliferation of cells at the lower end of the fused muellerian
    (paramesonephric) ducts and the vagina below the hymen from
    the urogenital sinus. The complete longitudinal vaginal septum
    and the double cervix found in this patient represents failure of
    fusion of the two paramesonephric ducts. When the cervix is
    duplicated there is usually a double uterus, of which one horn may
    be rudimentary. Alternatively, the uterus may contain an
    incomplete septum (subseptate) or may be heart-shaped (arcuate).
    The vaginal septum is commonly incomplete and there is
    frequently only a single cervix. Transverse vaginal septa may also
    be found; these are usually thin but may occasionally cause partial
    vaginal atresia. If an incomplete transverse septum develops high
    in the vagina it may resemble the cervix and cause confusion
    during labour.

2. Postmortem examinations have demonstrated that urogenital
    anomalies occur more frequently than those of any other system
    and are present in approximately 10% of women. Because of the
    close developmental association between the genital and urinary
    systems, it is not surprising that genital tract anomalies are
    frequently associated with abnormalities of the urinary tract. These
    include double and ectopic ureter, ectopic urethral orifice, etc.
    Paravaginal cysts arising from the remnant of the mesonephric
    (Gartner's) ducts may also be found. Rarely, there may be
    persistence of the urogenital (cloacal) sinus.

3. During labour, a longitudinal vaginal septum is usually pushed to
    one side by the descending head. It may occasionally cause delay
    in the descent of the presenting part, or even become lacerated
    and cause profuse bleeding at the time of delivery. Some
    obstetricians favour division of the septum either during
    pregnancy or as an interval procedure. Most would, however, elect
    to follow a conservative course and divide the septum during
    labour should this prove to be necessary. This patient laboured
    spontaneously at 42 weeks. Progress in the first stage of labour
    was normal, but the septum caused some soft tissue resistance in
    the second stage. An assisted delivery was therefore performed
    using a vacuum extractor (Ventouse). The septum was not divided
    and it did not tear.

4. When a vagina septum is associated with a uterine anomaly, fetal
    malpresentation is common. In this case, however, the lie
    remained longitudinal and the presentation cephalic through the
    last trimester. Examination of the uterine cavity after delivery
    suggested that it was of normal shape despite the presence of two
    cervices.

Obstetrics 33

A 32-year-old insulin-dependent diabetic was booked for hospital confinement at the end of the 8th week of her 3rd pregnancy. Her first had ended in a spontaneous miscarriage at 12 weeks gestation, but her second had progressed uneventfully to term with a spontaneous vaginal delivery of a 4.06 kg male infant. The present pregnancy was planned and she had already started to adjust her insulin dosage according to her blood glucose levels, as she had done in her previous pregnancy. Ultrasound scan confirmed the gestation and a detailed scan at 18 weeks showed no obvious fetal abnormality.

The pregnancy progressed uneventfully under the joint care of the obstetrician and physician, the fetal growth being monitored by monthly ultrasound scans. Blood glucose levels were all between 4.2 and 4.8 mmol/1 and weekly cardiotocograms from 32 weeks were normal. The 36-week ultrasound scan estimated fetal weight to be between 4 and 4.5 kg and examination of the patient's abdomen at 38 weeks confirmed engagement of the fetal head.

The patient went into spontaneous labour at 39 weeks and progressed to full dilatation in 8 hours. The head delivered spontaneously after a 35-minute second stage, but despite all the patient's and the midwives' efforts the shoulders would not deliver.

1. What is the management of shoulder dystocia?
2. How might shoulder dystocia be predicted?

1. Treatment should be swift and as gentle as possible under the circumstances. The patient should be put in the lithotomy position. In an emergency, this can be performed by turning her across the bed so that her perineum is just over the edge. Her legs can be held by assistants, one of whom should press down on the patient's abdomen just above the symphysis pubis. A substantial episiotomy should be performed and then the fetal head grasped firmly between the operator's hands and pressed down towards the perineum at the same time as applying traction to deliver the body. A finger can occasionally be inserted into the baby's axilla to provide additional traction. Once delivered, the baby should immediately be wrapped up and the umbilical cord cut. There will usually be a low Apgar score and skilled paediatric help should be sought rapidly.

   Occasionally the above manoeuvres will not be sufficient to deliver the baby. In this case, the step is to pass a hand posterior to the head (this is always easy to do as, by definition, the shoulders are held up above the pelvic brim) and rotate the posterior shoulder in the direction of least resistance until it lies below the symphysis pubis (a sort of reverse Lovset's manoeuvre). The shoulder can then be delivered by finger traction in the axilla. If the baby is still not far enough down, it may be necessary to repeat the manoeuvre. In the last resort, the arm may need to be broken in order to deliver it. This sounds dramatic, but healing is usually rapid without serious sequelae. Techniques whereby the head is pushed back into the uterus and the baby then delivered by caesarean section have been described, but this is not a technique of which the authors have any experience.

2. Shoulder dystocia should be anticipated in any delivery where the baby is likely to be larger than average, or the patient is smaller than average. Thus, any woman with a history of large babies or diabetes should be carefully assessed before delivery in order to estimate fetal size. Ultrasound scan measurement of the bisacromial diameter will provide some idea of the shoulder size and taken together with pelvimetry, clinical or radiographic, should help alert the obstetric team to the possibility of shoulder dystocia. However, many studies have shown that reliable prediction is difficult, and the only safe plan is, like boy scouts, always to 'be prepared' for the possibility.

Obstetrics 34

Following an uneventful pregnancy, a 29-year-old primigravida was delivered of a healthy 3.65 kg male infant by elective caesarean section in accordance with her hospital's policy for breech presentation. The operation was straightforward and the surgeon noted that the uterus had a midline septum.

Two years later the woman booked for antenatal care in her second pregnancy. Like the first, this pregnancy progressed uneventfully and when she was reviewed by the consultant at 38 weeks gestation the presentation was cephalic and the fetal head engaged. The patient was particularly keen to deliver vaginally and so it was decided to await the onset of labour and allow a trial of scar.

Labour began spontaneously at 40 weeks gestation. On admission to the labour ward the cervix was 4 cm dilated and well applied to the fetal head, which was in the occipitolateral position and 2 cm above the spines. Routine cardiotocography showed a baseline rate of 164 beats/minute with good variability.

Three hours after admission the fetal heart rate began decelerating irregularly and, while trying to relate them to uterine contractions, the registrar noted that these had become weaker and less frequent, although the patient was still complaining of strong abdominal pains. Vaginal examination was performed: the cervix was 5 cm dilated but only loosely applied to the fetal head.

1. Would you have allowed this patient a trial of scar?
2. What clinical features were suggestive of scar dehiscence?
3. What are the priorities of management?

1. The old saying, 'once a caesarean always a caesarean' has been disproved time and again for lower segment operations and many studies have confirmed that the incidence of scar rupture in subsequent labour is low (approximately 1 in 200), providing a degree of selection is made as to which women with previous caesarean section might be permitted a trial of scar. Thus, women of particularly short stature, pregnancies with malpresentation, large fetuses, or previous cephalopelvic disproportion with a normal size infant might not be suitable cases for vaginal delivery. In this particular case there were no obvious contraindications to trial of scar — the previously noted septate uterus does not necessarily preclude successful vaginal delivery. Nevertheless, and however unusual it may be, scar dehiscence is possible in any trial of scar and therefore the labour must be conducted in a unit where there are facilities for resuscitation and emergency repeat caesarean section.

2. The classical signs of uterine rupture do not as a rule appear in scar dehiscence though many features may be similar. Scar dehiscence is often painless and may only be detected when the patient is delivered by caesarean section, perhaps for failure to progress, or even in patients having elective repeat caesarean section. Similarly, bleeding is not usually a feature since the old scar is relatively avascular, though the appearance of fresh vaginal bleeding during a trial of scar should be taken seriously. Cessation of contractions and changes in the fetal heart rate are, however, strongly suggestive of scar dehiscence and must always be acted upon promptly. Action will nearly always need to be repeat caesarean section; attempts to assess fetal condition by fetal blood sampling introduce dangerous delay and, in any case, normal fetal acid–base balance does not preclude a dangerous uterine scar rupture.

3. The most important aspect of the management of scar dehiscence is to anticipate it and so an intravenous line should be inserted at the onset of labour and blood should be crossmatched as a precaution. Cardiotocography allows continuous fetal monitoring and regular vaginal examinations confirm that labour is progressing and that the fetal head is descending. If scar rupture is suspected, caesarean section should be performed without delay, preferably by an experienced surgeon. Once the baby has been delivered the uterus must be inspected carefully and the degree of damage from the dehiscence assessed: in most cases only the scar will have dehisced, but occasionally the tear will have extended into previously uninvolved myometrium. Providing bleeding can be controlled, the scar can be repaired in the usual way, but if there is any doubt, then hysterectomy should be considered.

A 29-year-old woman who had been sterilised by laparoscopic tubal diathermy after the delivery of her second child in her previous marriage requested reversal of sterilisation. The marriage had ended in divorce and she had remarried 2 years later. Her present husband had no children of his own.

A postcoital test performed on the 13th day of the menstrual cycle showed large numbers of actively motile sperm and so a diagnostic laparoscopy was performed to assess the feasibility of reversal. Sadly, the tubes were almost completely destroyed by the diathermy, making the prospects for successful reversal extremely low and the couple were advised accordingly. Having discussed the situation fully they opted for in vitro fertilisation and this was successful on the first attempt. Ultrasound scan at 8 weeks gestation showed the presence of at least 3 fetuses and a repeat scan 4 weeks later confirmed quadruplets.

During the subsequent 12 weeks the woman was seen fortnightly in the antenatal clinic and the uterus was noted to be enlarging rapidly: by 24 weeks the fundal size was equivalent to a term pregnancy and serial scans confirmed that all 4 fetuses were growing well. Because the patient was so uncomfortable she was admitted to hospital at the beginning of the 25th week for rest. Three days later she began draining clear fluid per vaginam.

1. How would you confirm that the membranes had ruptured?
2. Could any steps have been taken to reduce the risk of preterm labour?
3. How would you deliver the patient?

1. The traditional methods of diagnosing premature rupture of membranes rely on a combination of history, speculum visualisation of liquor in the vagina and the characteristic smell of liquor. Nitrazine stick testing is much less reliable than is often assumed and is prone to false positive results (it is only a measure of pH, nitrazine turning from orange to black at pHs above 6.7 — it is not a specific test for the presence of liquor). A more reliable approach is to use ultrasound to investigate the volume of amniotic fluid remaining in the uterus; demonstration of a normal liquor volume indicates a good prognosis, even if liquor appears to be draining.

2. There is no reliable method of preventing preterm labour in multiple pregnancies and tocolytics such as salbutamol and ritodrine will, at best, only delay delivery for a short time. Cervical sutures enjoyed a brief period of popularity, but there is no evidence in relation to multiple pregnancy that they are any more effective than bed rest or tocolysis. A much more controversial method of reducing the risk of preterm labour is to reduce the number of fetuses by selective fetocide. This is performed before the end of the first trimester, usually by inserting a fine needle into the fetal heart under ultrasound control. Quite clearly, the procedure carries risks as well as major moral and ethical implications and should only be performed where all parties concerned are in agreement.

3. Although caesarean section seems the obvious choice as the preferred mode of delivery, there are risks to the mother and several studies have failed to show an improvement in fetal outcome at this gestation. The most important aspect of management is to have adequate help at delivery and this entails a large number of people. There should be a paediatrician, a paediatric trained nurse, an incubator and sufficient resuscitation equipment for each baby. Anyone who has taken part in such highly organised deliveries will attest to the sheer amount of space required!

Obstetrics 36

A 26-year-old primigravida was found to have a breech presentation at her routine 38-week clinic visit. Since she was of average build and height and the fetal weight was estimated clinically to be no more than 3 kg, it was decided that a vaginal delivery could be attempted.

Exactly 1 week later she went into spontaneous labour. Vaginal examination on admission to hospital revealed a fully effaced cervix dilated to 5 cm. The presenting part was a breech and was about 1 cm above the spines. A fetal electrode was fixed to the breech and a normal cardiotocogram obtained. An epidural was inserted for analgesia and labour allowed to continue.

Full dilatation was reached 6 hours after admission and the woman was therefore encouraged to bear down with each contraction. She pushed well, despite being unable to feel her contractions because of a good epidural block, but after 2 hours there had been virtually no descent of the presenting part. A caesarean section was performed under epidural and a healthy 3.57 kg male infant delivered.

1. Should she have had pelvimetry?
2. Would she have been more likely to deliver if she had not had an epidural?
3. Would you have used oxytocin to improve the contractions and help descent of the presenting part in the second stage?
4. Was the labour a waste of time?

1. Many studies have failed to show a convincing benefit from measures of pelvic size using X-ray pelvimetry. This is because prediction of mode of delivery also requires an accurate knowledge of fetal size and, at present, ultrasound estimates have a minimum 15% uncertainty (e.g. an estimated fetal weight of 3.4 kg is consistent with a true weight of 2.9 kg or 3.9 kg). However, pelvimetry is still commonly performed for medicolegal reasons.

   Far more important for clinical management is progress in labour and descent of the breech in the second stage. The old admonition 'never touch the breech until it climbs the perineum' is probably the most valuable aid to safe management of breech delivery. Provided that labour in such a case is conducted in a hospital with experienced staff and facilities for caesarean section, it is probably unnecessary to perform X-ray pelvimetry.

2. There is no evidence that epidural analgesia will make vaginal delivery less likely.

3. If the contractions are normal and cervical dilatation reasonably rapid, there is little to be gained by using oxytocin and it may actually be harmful if it causes uterine hyperstimulation. If the contractions are hypotonic, then oxytocin is probably of value, but an intrauterine catheter should be used to monitor the contractions if possible.

4. Allowing this lady to labour may not have achieved a vaginal delivery in this pregnancy, but it will increase her chances of a successful vaginal delivery in her next one.

Obstetrics 37

A 29-year-old youth worker presented herself at the hospital antenatal clinic at about 17 weeks gestation requesting booking for antenatal care and confinement. She was unmarried, but in a stable relationship. She and her partner had recently moved into the area. They had not yet registered with a local general practitioner, but according to the woman she had always been perfectly well. She brought with her a birth plan detailing her feelings about, and wishes for, the management of her pregnancy. These included a request for an undertaking from the hospital staff that no vaginal examination was to be performed until she was in labour. She declined a cervical smear on the grounds that one taken by her previous general practitioner several months earlier had been normal. Her wishes were respected and arrangements were made to see her monthly until the 28th week of pregnancy.

Three weeks later, the senior midwife in the antenatal clinic received a telephone call from the patient's previous general practitioner. It transpired that the patient had had a number of abnormal cervical smears over the previous two years, the most recent showing the presence of severely dyskaryotic cells. The patient had been referred to the local hospital for colposcopy but had failed to keep her appointment: it was only when the general practitioner was notified of this several weeks later and tried to contact the woman that he had discovered from her mother — who was unaware of her daughter's abnormal smears — that she had moved away and was pregnant. He was also able to find out from her which hospital she was booked at.

The subject was raised with the patient when she attended the antenatal clinic the following week. In a tearful interview she confessed that she was certain she would be told she would have to have a hysterectomy for her abnormal smear and had therefore decided that she would ignore the abnormal smears and get pregnant.

1. Would you repeat the smear, or go straight to colposcopy and biopsy?
2. If the diagnosis was as CIN II, when and how would you deliver the baby?
3. If the diagnosis was microinvasion less than 2 mm, would you :
   (i)   deliver immediately and proceed to a Wertheim hysterectomy
   (ii) perform a cone biopsy
   (iii) wait until 32 weeks gestation, deliver the baby by caesarean section and perform a cone biopsy 6 weeks later?

1. The most important step in the management of this case is counselling and education. The patient should immediately be reassured that, provided this is still a precancerous lesion, the pregnancy can be allowed to continue and that the vast majority of cases can be treated without hysterectomy.

   From a medical point of view, the next step is colposcopy, preferably preceded immediately by a cervical smear. It is essential that the colposcopy is done by an experienced colposcopist since it is not always easy to see the cervix clearly in pregnancy and the colposcopic appearances are often altered. In many cases the assessment may be made by cytology and colposcopy alone, but if there is any doubt a biopsy should be performed. If the lesion is small a colposcopically directed biopsy may be taken and the site cauterised with a 'cold' coagulator. In this case the patient should be admitted for 24 hours, or until the bleeding has settled.

2. CIN alone may simply be observed through the pregnancy with colposcopy at 32–34 weeks to exclude progression to invasive disease (colposcopy at later stages in the third trimester is more difficult because of the increasingly lax vaginal walls preventing a good view of the cervix). A vaginal delivery is permissible unless there are obstetric contraindications. Repeat colposcopy is then performed about 6 weeks after delivery and the appropriate treatment given.

3. If microinvasion is suspected from the colposcopic appearances, loop excision or cone biopsy should be performed despite the risks to the pregnancy. Some authorities will allow a subsequent vaginal delivery in a case where there is only very early microinvasion completely removed by the cone: others consider this an indication for caesarean section because vaginal delivery predisposes to dissemination of maligant cells into the lymphatics and blood vessels.

   In invasive disease the pregnancy must be terminated and the patient treated with surgery and/or radiotherapy. If the pregnancy is sufficiently advanced, a caesarean section can be performed but if not the fetus must be sacrificed.

   In this particular case CIN III was found and the patient allowed to have a normal delivery. The lesion was treated 6 weeks postpartum by laser ablation.

Obstetrics 38

A 22-year-old Irish woman booked at 17 weeks gestation in her third
pregnancy. Her two previous pregnancies had been completely
normal and had ended in spontaneous vaginal deliveries. The babies
were both male, weighing 2.9 kg and 2.75 kg at 42 and 41 weeks
respectively. The present pregnancy was unplanned, but nevertheless
welcome, and the patient was certain of the date of her last menstrual
period. The only problem so far in this pregnancy was that there had
been some vaginal bleeding in the 12th week, but this had settled
after 2 days of resting in bed. She smoked 20–25 cigarettes per day
and drank about 2 units of alcohol each week.

Booking blood pressure was 130/80, her urine was clear and fundal
size was equal to the period of amenorrhoea. Blood was taken for
haemoglobin estimation, grouping and antibody screen and serum
alpha-fetoprotein level and the patient asked to attend her general
practitioner for shared antenatal care until she was 34 weeks
pregnant. One week later the laboratory notified the hospital antenatal
clinic sister that the patient's serum alpha-fetoprotein level was 120
ku/l (the median x 2.5 at this gestation is 88 ku/l).

1. What is alpha-fetoprotein?
2. What are the possible causes of an elevated alpha-fetoprotein
   level?
3. What further steps in management are required?

1. Alpha-fetoprotein is fetal albumin. It is found in small amounts in both amniotic fluid and maternal serum in normal pregnancies, the quantity being related to the gestation and generally rising until about the 22nd week before falling again to a very low level at term.

2. It therefore follows that if the dates are wrong and the pregnancy is more advanced than originally thought, the alpha-fetoprotein level will appear to be raised. It will also be raised in multiple pregnancy and it may be elevated when there has been fetomaternal haemorrhage, such as may occur in a threatened abortion. It is incorrect, therefore, to assume automatically that the raised level indicates a break in the fetal skin, such as occurs in open neural tube defects and exomphalos. In many women the raised level simply represents the extreme end of the normal population distribution.

3. If the serum alpha-fetoprotein is found to be raised, it is essential to confirm the gestational age of the fetus and to exclude multiple pregnancy, though it should be borne in mind that a neural tube defect can occur in one or more fetuses in a multiple pregnancy. Before embarking on any further investigation it is essential to counsel the patient so that she is fully aware of its significance. A high-resolution ultrasound scan should then be performed with detailed attention being paid to the fetal spine and abdomen. In the absence of such ultrasound facilities, or if there is still doubt, the patient should be offered amniocentesis to determine the amniotic fluid level of alpha-fetoprotein and acetylcholinesterase (released from any exposed nervous tissue), the latter being done because any bloodstaining of the amniotic fluid sample with fetal blood will give a falsely elevated alpha-fetoprotein level but will not affect the acetylcholinesterase level.

   If no cause for the raised level can be found, the pregnancy should still be closely monitored because of the association between raised serum alpha-fetoprotein levels in the second trimester and intrauterine growth retardation in later pregnancy (this may be due to the link both have with heavy maternal cigarette smoking).

   In this particular case the patient was found on detailed ultrasound scan to have a twin pregnancy with two normal fetuses.

Obstetrics 39

A 20-year-old Asian woman booked at the antenatal clinic in a district general hospital with a level 2 special care baby unit (SCBU) at 17 weeks gestation in her second pregnancy. Her first pregnancy had ended at about 14 weeks gestation as a miscarriage. An evacuation of retained products was performed and she conceived again soon afterwards.

On examination she was noted to be in good health, normotensive and with a fundal height equivalent to dates. Urinalysis was clear. Routine ultrasound scan confirmed that the biparietal diameter of the fetal head was equivalent to dates, but the placenta was seen to be situated anteriorly and low lying, covering the internal os. A repeat scan at 30 weeks gestation showed that the placenta was still overlying the internal os and a further scan was arranged for 32 weeks gestation. Three days before this, however, she was admitted as an emergency having passed approximately one cupful of blood clot vaginally following several hours of dull lower abdominal pain. Her general condition was satisfactory with a pulse of 80 beats per minute and a blood pressure of 130/80 mmHg. The fundus felt equivalent to dates, the fetus could be easily palpated and was found to be in cephalic presentation with 5/5 palpable per abdomen. Cardiotocography showed a normal reactive pattern.

The patient was kept in hospital under observation and 4 hours later had a further bleed, this time accompanied by severe abdominal pain. Her pulse was 100 beats/minute, blood pressure 100/60 mmHg and she could feel contractions distinct from the lower abdominal pain. The cardiotocogram showed a fetal heart rate pattern with a baseline rate of 179 beats per minute with no accelerations or decelerations and reduced baseline variability. The contraction channel showed small contractions occurring every minute.

1. What is the most likely cause of the bleeding?
2. How could this be confirmed?
3. How would you deliver her?
4. Where would you deliver her?

1. Antepartum haemorrhage is traditionally divided into three groups: bleeding from a normally situated placenta, bleeding from an abnormally situated placenta and bleeding from other sites. The placenta in this particular case was known to be low lying and initially it could reasonably be assumed that the bleeding was due to placenta praevia. However, the onset of labour and severe lower abdominal pain, together with the slight deterioration in maternal condition, is suggestive of placental abruption: there is, after all, no reason why an abnormally situated placenta should not be associated with abruption and retroplacental bleeding.

2. An important aid in the diagnosis of antepartum haemorrhage is ultrasound scanning, which will localise the placenta. Occasionally it can also reveal blood clot between the placenta and the uterine wall. Things were not so simple in this particular case, however, because no blood clot could be seen within the uterine cavity. The abruption was of the revealed type, the clot lying in the vagina and presumably not expelled because the patient had been kept in the recumbent position and not examined vaginally because of the known low-lying placenta.

   An important aspect of the diagnosis in this case is the CTG pattern. The small frequent contractions are typical of abruptio placentae and are probably due to massive prostaglandin release secondary to decidual disruption. The lack of accelerations and the loss of variability suggest early fetal hypoxia; the next stage would be the appearance of shallow late decelerations which are sometimes mistaken for baseline variability because the contractions are so frequent.

3. Given that the placenta was clearly identified as low-lying, and there is strong evidence of abruption, delivery by caesarean section is indicated. In the absence of ultrasound facilities, this would have to be preceded by examination in a fully prepared operating theatre ready for caesarean section if the placenta was encountered.

4. Because of the gestation, the neonate would almost certainly require neonatal intensive care facilities, something not available in a level 2 special care unit. Nevertheless, it is essential to take into account not just the needs of the baby but also those of the mother. In a situation such as this case, there is every possibility that the bleeding might become worse and the mother develop shock, which would naturally be difficult to manage in a moving ambulance.

   Ideally, this case should be managed in a unit with facilities for both mother and baby but this is not always possible, so the condition of both mother and fetus must be carefully considered before any transfer is made. The whole episode described above occurred in a district general hospital provided with only limited special care baby unit facilities. Intrauterine transfer was clearly contraindicated because of the mother's condition and the limited facilities in the hospital were already fully extended. Immediately after delivery, therefore, the neonate was transferred to the nearest available unit with neonatal intensive care, some 40 miles away. Thanks to absence of road traffic and a skilled neonatal care team, the baby survived, though the mother was only able to be reunited with her child 5 days later.

Obstetrics 40

A 26-year-old housewife was referred to the antenatal clinic for booking in her third pregnancy. Her two previous pregnancies had ended in a first trimester therapeutic termination and subsequently a miscarriage at 10 weeks gestation. She gave no significant family history and was in good health. She smoked 20 cigarettes per day. Her dates were somewhat uncertain, but a scan made her 12 weeks at the time of booking. A singleton normal fetus was identified and serum alpha-fetoprotein estimation at 17 weeks was normal.

She attended the antenatal clinic regularly and the pregnancy progressed uneventfully until the 36th week visit, when it was noted that the fundal size was larger than expected, fetal parts were difficult to palpate and there was an excess of liquor. The fetal heart was easily audible, but at a rate of 200 beats per minute. A cardiotocograph tracing confirmed the high rate and showed some decreased baseline variability. There were no decelerations of the fetal heart rate, but the tracing was non-reactive.

The patient was advised to stay in hospital for further monitoring, but declined, only to be admitted some 12 hours later in strong labour following spontaneous rupture of membranes. She felt well in herself and was apyrexial with a blood pressure of 120/85 and pulse rate of 80 beats per minute. Clear liquor was draining vaginally and cervical dilatation was 6 cm. A fetal scalp electrode was applied and the CTG showed a baseline rate of 200 beats per minute with minimal variability and deep variable decelerations. Fetal scalp blood pH was 7.35 on two occasions over the next hour, with good samples having been obtained and pH machine calibration having been checked. By this time the cervix was 9 cm dilated and the position of the head was occipito-anterior.

1. What could account for the abnormal CTG pattern in the absence of hypoxia or acidosis?
2. How could the abnormal pattern have been investigated further before the onset of labour?
3. Would you deliver the baby by caesarean section at this point?
4. If not, why not?

1. A baseline tachycardia with variable decelerations may be due to a number of causes, including cord compression and hypoxia. This pattern may also be due to a congenital cardiac anomaly.

2. The abnormal CTG pattern could have been investigated further by performing a cardiac scan to exclude a congenital malformation, and a Doppler scan may have shown an abnormal waveform consistent with a cardiac anomaly. Both, however, require expert ultrasonographers to identify and then interpret the findings.

3. When a pattern like this occurs in labour, simple measures such as turning the patient on her side should be instituted without delay. If the pattern persists, and delivery is not imminent, then scalp blood pH should be measured: if this is below 7.25 it indicates acidosis and the fetus should be delivered as soon as possible. If the pH is above this level, however, the patient can be managed more conservatively, but the pH should be checked at half-hourly intervals for as long as the trace abnormality persists.

4. If the pH level had been below 7.25, the baby should have been delivered by caesarean section, irrespective of cervical dilatation, to avoid the added insult of forceps delivery; the added danger from forceps is particularly great if rotation is required.

   Full dilatation occurred shortly after the second fetal blood sample was taken and therefore an elective low forceps (non-rotational) was performed to expedite the second stage. Despite active resuscitation for 15 minutes, the fetus failed to show any signs of life. The baby, a male, appeared externally normal, but there were only two vessels in the umbilical cord. Autopsy subsequently showed multiple cardiac abnormalities which included an absent atrial septum. The liver was much enlarged, consistent with fetal cardiac failure.

Obstetrics 41

A 22-year-old woman attended the hospital antenatal booking clinic in the 8th week of her second pregnancy. Her first pregnancy had ended 18 months earlier in a spontaneous vaginal delivery of a healthy male infant weighing 3.15 kg, at 40 weeks gestation. This second pregnancy was planned and had been conceived 4 months after stopping a progesterone-only contraceptive pill.

There was nothing untoward in her history but she reported feeling nauseous most mornings. Her breasts were tender and she had begun to gain weight. Examination revealed a healthy looking young woman with a blood pressure of 110/70, a pulse rate of 70 beats per minute, no obvious pallor and increasing pigmentation aound the nipples. There were no masses palpable per abdomen and urinalysis was clear. Vaginal examination was not performed. The woman was given supplementary iron and folic acid and asked to see her general practitioner monthly for the next 2 months before attending the hospital antenatal clinic at 17 weeks gestation for a routine ultrasound scan and serum alpha-fetoprotein estimation.

At this visit the woman reported that she had been feeling well and her only concern was that four weeks previously she had noticed slight vaginal bleeding, which settled after bedrest. She was happy to report that her nausea had settled shortly after this and her breasts no longer tingled. On examination the findings were as before, but the uterus could be palpated just above the symphysis pubis. She was then directed to the ultrasound department for her prearranged scan and asked to return to the clinic as soon as it had been performed. Less than an hour later she was brought back to the clinic in a distraught state.

1. What did the ultrasound scan show?
2. How do the clinical findings tie in with this result?
3. How would you manage the situation subsequently?

1. The ultrasound scan showed a collapsed gestation sac with nothing more than disorganised echoes within it. The appearances were compatible with a missed abortion.

2. Taken individually, light vaginal bleeding in the 12th week, cessation of nausea and breast tenderness and a uterus smaller than dates are often insignificant. Taken together, however, they are strongly suggestive that the pregnancy is no longer viable and a missed abortion is a likely finding.

3. In a situation such as this, the most important factor is a sympathetic approach to the patient. An evacuation of retained products of conception may be required, but it is not an emergency procedure and wherever possible the patient should be given an opportunity to come to terms with the situation and arrange for her family and friends to be told. If the gestation sac is small (less than 2 cm in diameter) spontaneous miscarriage may occur and if this appears to be complete, evacuation may not be necessary. If evacuation is necessary, admission can be delayed for several days, though in practice most women are keen to come in within 24 hours. If she still has any difficulty accepting the fact that the pregnancy is not progressing normally, a repeat ultrasound scan should be performed. Products of conception should always be sent for histological confirmation and the patient's rhesus blood grouping checked so that anti-D immunoglobulin can be given if required.

   Each gynaecologist will have his or her own opinion as to how long a woman in this situation should wait before trying for another pregnancy. The incidence of further miscarriage and placenta praevia has been reported to be slightly increased if conception occurs within three months and, in practice, most couples elect to wait some months before trying again. However, couples should be reassured that if conception occurs before this time the pregnancy is likely to be successful and uncomplicated. An early ultrasound scan in the next pregnancy with repeats at 12 and 16 weeks will make no difference to the pregnancy outcome, but are enormously reassuring to the patient.

Obstetrics 42

A 26-year-old nulliparous woman was admitted to the labour ward in spontaneous labour at 41 weeks gestation following an uneventful pregnancy. Her membranes had ruptured spontaneously several hours earlier and uterine contractions were occurring once every 10 minutes. Abdominal palpation confirmed a term-sized singleton fetus in cephalic presentation with three-fifths of the head palpable. On vaginal examination the cervix was fully effaced, 3 cm dilated and well applied to the presenting part which was just above the level of the ischial spines and in transverse position. The fetal heart rate was regular at 135–140 beats per minute.

Over the next 4 hours the contractions became stronger and more frequent and on vaginal examination the cervix had dilated to 6 cm. The fetal head was still just above the ischial spines, the occiput directly on the right. Epidural analgesia was requested and provided with good effect, but when progress was reassessed 4 hours later the cervix had only dilated to 7 cm and the fetal head was still right occipito-transverse, poorly flexed and at the level of the spines. An oxytocin infusion was set up and continuous fetal heart rate monitoring started using a scalp electrode.

Two hours later the cardiotocograph trace began registering decelerations, initially during contractions, but later occurring after them. After one particularly severe deceleration starting 30 seconds after the contraction peak, falling to 60 beats per minute and then rising slowly over the subsequent 2 minutes, vaginal examination was performed and revealed full dilatation with fetal position still deflexed right occcipito-transverse and just below the level of the spines. There was a small amount of fresh meconium present in the liquor.

1. Expeditious delivery is clearly indicated; what alternatives are open to you?
2. Before deciding which route to choose, what additional information would you require?
3. With hindsight, how might this situation have been avoided?

1. The baby can be delivered abdominally by caesarean section, or vaginally after rotating the head into the occipito-anterior or, less advisably, the occipito-posterior position. Rotation can be accomplished by the use of appropriate forceps, by Ventouse and manually.

2. Additional information required must include both the amount of fetal head palpable per abdomen and the fetal blood pH because of the risks to the baby of a rotation forceps delivery in the presence of the cerebral oedema, which accompanies acidosis. Thus, if one-fifth or more of the fetal head is palpable per abdomen, delivery should be by caesarean section, irrespective of the pH. If the fetal head is no longer palpable per abdomen and the pH is greater than 7.25, vaginal delivery could be attempted by rotation of the fetal head. The method of rotation will largely depend on the experience of the operator. Manual rotation followed by forceps lift-out generally requires the least experience, whilst forceps rotation and delivery requires the most experience. In all cases, adequate analgesia must be provided using pudendal block, epidural and (rarely) general anaesthesia, and ideally should be performed in theatre with facilities for caesarean section if required.

   If the pH is below 7.25, the baby should be delivered by caesarean section: the delay likely to be experienced is less important than avoiding rotational forceps in the presence of acidosis and cerebral oedema.

3. In the face of relative disproportion, such as with a transverse position, nulliparae will often respond by developing inco-ordinate uterine action. This is most easily diagnosed by a slowing down in the rate of cervical dilatation at around 6–7 cm. Having diagnosed a transverse position at an early stage in this patient's labour, it might have been appropriate to start an oxytocic infusion once the head had failed to rotate by the second vaginal examination. An alternative approach might have been to encourage the patient to walk about as much as possible, since the movement of the pelvis sometimes encourages the head to rotate spontaneously.

Obstetrics 43

A 24-year-old married Caucasian woman presented herself at the casualty department of a hospital complaining of a painful and swollen left leg. She was just over 26 weeks pregnant in her second pregnancy, the first having ended in a spontaneous miscarriage at 10 weeks gestation approximately 2 years earlier. In the interim she had taken the combined oral contraceptive pill.

The present pregnancy had been uneventful until 5 days earlier when she developed swelling of the left ankle. This had become progressively worse over the subsequent few days, despite bed rest, and had extended to involve the whole leg. It had gradually become painful over the course of the day before she came to the hospital. The pain was initially restricted to the thigh and groin but soon affected the whole left leg. She was otherwise well and had no cough, chest pain or shortness of breath.

On examination, the left leg was swollen, discoloured and markedly tender to touch. Passive movement was severely restricted and flexing the ankle, knee or thigh provoked extreme pain. The uterine size corresponded to dates and fetal movements had remained normal throughout.

1. What is the diagnosis?
2. What further investigations would you perform?
3. How would you treat this condition?

1. The most likely diagnosis is thrombosis of the major veins of the left leg. Although thrombosis and embolism are much more common in the puerperium than in pregnancy, they appear to be more dangerous in the latter and have been associated with a higher maternal mortality than those occurring in the puerperium. This may be because embolism is more likely to occur in pregnancy, but it may also be because of failure to diagnose and treat thrombosis soon enough.

2. The simplest diagnostic test for suspected thrombosis involves the use of ultrasound. A standard Doppler machine is used to detect the flow, or absence thereof, in the veins of the popliteal fossa and in the groin. Absent sounds are highly suggestive of thrombosis. Phlebography may be helpful, but it is a painful procedure requiring a fair degree of skill to perform and interpret. Radioactive imaging is contraindicated in pregnancy.

3. Treatment always involves admission to hospital, bed rest and anticoagulation. Some authorities suggest the use of compression stockings to prevent further thrombus formation.
   Anticoagulation is initiated with intravenous heparin, preferably given by slow infusion of 40000 units over 24 hours, aiming to achieve a level of 0.6–1.0 units per ml using the protamine sulphate neutralisation test. Once the pain settles, the patient is encouraged to move about, but the heparin is continued. Other anticoagulants such as warfarin may be used, but in pregnancy after 26 weeks it is probably safer to continue with heparin, given subcutaneously by the patient herself, because it can easily be reversed with protamine sulphate should the need arise.

Obstetrics 44

A 22-year-old primigravida was admitted to the labour ward at 39 weeks gestation with spontaneous rupture of her membranes after an uneventful pregnancy. On arrival she was noted to be draining clear liquor, but was only having weak contractions once every 20 minutes. The cervix was still about 2 centimetres long and just admitted a fingertip. The fetal heart was auscultated with a Pinard stethoscope and the rate found to be 146 beats per minute and regular. The woman was encouraged to walk about as she wished until contractions became established.

Fourteen hours and a good sleep later, uterine contractions were still weak and irregular, though she continued to drain clear liquor. Her general condition was good, she was apyrexial and the fetal heart rate remained normal. Vaginal examination confirmed that there had been no change in cervical dilatation. It was therefore decided that labour should be induced with an oxytocic infusion. Six hours later the cervix was effaced, moderately well applied to the presenting part and about 5 cm dilated. An epidural was inserted for analgesia and the oxytocin infusion continued.

Full dilatation was reached 11 hours after the infusion was begun and after pushing for 90 minutes a forceps lift-out was performed for 'maternal exhaustion'. Syntometrine (syntocinon 5 units and ergometrine 0.5 mg) was given intramuscularly with the delivery of the anterior shoulder. After waiting for signs of separation, the placenta was delivered by continuous cord traction. Unfortunately, this was followed by a rapid haemorrhage of almost a litre of blood.

1. What aspect of the labour might have contributed to the postpartum haemorrhage (PPH)?
2. How could the delivery and third stage have been managed differently?
3. The patient's haemoglobin on the third day after delivery was 8.6 g/dl. What would you advise?

1. Prolonged oxytocic infusion often predisposes to uterine atony and hence postpartum haemorrhage.

2. In cases such as this the oxytocin infusion rate should be increased immediately following delivery and syntometrine is often better given as the fetal head is delivered, rather than waiting for the anterior shoulder. If there is any sign of atony, the uterus should be compressed bimanually until a further dose of ergometrine is given and/or the uterus contracts.

3. The traditional response to a haemoglobin this low is blood transfusion and there is no doubt that women in this situation feel very much better for it, particularly if they intend to breast feed. Nevertheless, there is a growing resistance to transfusion on the part of the public because of the perceived risk of transmission of infectious diseases (particularly HIV) and many women will decline transfusion unless 'absolutely necessary'. In such situations the value of transfusion should be compared to the disadvantages, especially the tiredness and lethargy that may be experienced and the woman herself given the final say. If transfusion is refused, iron supplements should be commenced immediately and continued until the haemoglobin level rises to normal.

Obstetrics 45

After many years of involuntary infertility, a 38-year-old woman conceived spontaneously and was referred to her local hospital for antenatal care and confinement. She was seen in the clinic at the beginning of the 13th week of pregnancy and found to be well. The uterus was just palpable above the symphysis pubis and gentle bimanual examination at the same time as performing a routine cervical smear confirmed the uterine size to be equivalent to dates. Genetic counselling was offered in view of her age and arrangements made to see her in the 16th week of pregnancy for ultrasound scan and amniocentesis.

The scan confirmed the presence of a viable fetus of size equivalent to dates. The placenta was mostly fundal but extended anteriorly towards the cervix. A number of fibroids were noted, the largest of which was about 4 cm in diameter and situated in the anterior wall of the uterus. Amniocentesis was performed under ultrasound control, the needle being inserted through the uterus about 2 cm below the lowest part of the placenta and just above the fibroid. Fifteen millilitres of clear liquor was obtained and sent for chromosome analysis. The patient was allowed home after 2 hours and a repeat scan to confirm that the fetus was still alive.

Over the subsequent few weeks the woman experienced occasional lower abdominal cramps, which she ignored since they subsided with bed rest and fetal movements were by now plentiful.

She was admitted to hospital as an emergency at 24 weeks gestation with progressively worsening colicky lower abdominal pain, nausea and vomiting. She was not shocked, but her pulse rate was 90 per minute, her blood pressure 130/90 and her temperature 39°C. Palpation provoked guarding and rigidity, which were most marked over the lower abdomen making full palpation of the uterus difficult, but the fundal size was equivalent to dates. An ultrasound scan was performed with some difficulty because of her abdominal tenderness. The placenta appeared normal with no evidence of abruption, there was no hydramnios and the fetus was active. The anterior wall fibroid was less obvious, but still present and it was noted that the area of maximal tenderness was over the fibroid.

1. What is the most likely diagnosis?
2. How should she be treated?

1. The differential diagnosis includes all the usual conditions that might cause an acute abdomen, but in this particular case the most likely diagnosis is fibroid degeneration. Placental abruption or infarction may produce severe pain, but are unlikely to be associated with pyrexia. Appendicitis is usually associated with greater constitutional disturbance and is unlikely when the pain is central and most marked over the uterus. Uterine bleeding following amniocentesis could present in this way, but it would be unlikely to occur after this length of time.

   Although fibroids will often flatten out and become indistinct during pregnancy they can still undergo degeneration, the commonest form of which is necrobiosis or 'red' degeneration, so-called because of the haemorrhagic appearance of the fibroid if sectioned histologically. The pain may be due to ischaemia in the intramural portion of the fibroid or involvement of the visceral peritoneum in the subserous portion.

2. Management is conservative with bed rest and adequate analgesia for the pain. The symptoms will usually subside in 10–14 days and the patient can be reassured that the pregnancy is unlikely to be affected. Surgery is contraindicated because of the risk of severe haemorrhage and of precipitating preterm labour. The longer term management should include review at 6–8 weeks postpartum and 6–12 months later to reassess the size of the fibroids. Provided they are asymptomatic in terms of menstrual problems, or in relation to their size, no further treatment is required.

A 28-year-old Negro West Indian woman attended the accident and emergency department, following a fall. Examination revealed no serious trauma, but a mass arising from the pelvis extending to just above the umbilicus. She was very vague about the timing of her last menstrual period, but a scan showed a fetus with a BPD on the mean for 25 weeks. Blood was taken for the routine booking investigations and she was given an appointment for the antenatal clinic. However, she failed to attend and the community midwives discovered that she had moved from the address given on her visit to the accident and emergency department. Enquiries revealed that she had an active court injunction against a male registered at the same address, the grounds being violence. It appeared that he was likely to be the father of her fetus.

The booking investigations were all normal (Hb 11.2 g/dl, sickle negative, blood group A +ve, hep.B antibody titre negative, rubella immune), but her VDRL was positive at a titre of 1 in 256 and both the TPHA and FTA were strongly positive (+++).

She was readmitted 7 weeks later through casualty, at 6.30 in the morning. She had been having regular pains every 4 minutes since 02.00 hours. On examination she was 4 cm dilated; a cardiotocogram was normal. No attempt was made to stop labour, and she gave birth 4 hours later to a female infant weighing 2.1 kg. Apgar scores were 4 at 1 minute, 7 at 5 minutes, and 9 at 10 minutes. The placenta weighed 750 g.

1. What do the initials VDRL, TPHA and FTA stand for, and what do they signify?
2. What treatment would you give to mother and baby?
3. What might happen to the baby if you did not treat it?
4. What is the significance of the placental weight?

1. The initials stand for the venereal disease research laboratory test, the treponema pallidum haemagglutination assay, and the fluorescent treponema antibody (absorption) test. They are all tests for syphilis. The VDRL test is non-specific and can be positive, even if the woman does not have syphilis, for example due to the anamnestic antibody response of pregnancy itself, viral infections, drug addiction, and autoimmune diseases such as systemic lupus erythematosus. The reason it is performed is that, if it is strongly positive it indicates a recent infection, while following old treated infections it becomes negative. However, a negative result is not a guarantee that treatment has been effective. The other two tests (TPHA, FTA) usually remain positive for life and are very specific, although the TPHA is occasionally positive in infectious mononucleosis. All three tests are positive following treponemal infection with yaws, which is the main differential diagnosis in women from the West Indies, South America, or Equatorial Africa.

2. The mother should be treated with 1 mega unit of benzylpenicillin 8-hourly for 5 days, followed by 1 mega unit of aqueous procaine penicillin daily for 10 days. If she is allergic to penicillin, erythromycin 500 mg orally 4 times daily for 21 days is sufficient, although compliance is often a problem in women such as the one described above if they are not in hospital. The newborn should be treated with intramuscular penicillin at a dose of 50000 units /kg body weight, for 15 days. The baby should be followed up for at least 2 years and observed for any signs of relapse. Treatment of both mother and baby can be monitored by weekly VDRL estimations, which should fall steadily. Once a low level has been achieved, a check VDRL every 3 months will guard against recrudescence; a 4-fold rise in titre indicates the need for a repeat course of treatment.

3. Untreated, the baby will develop the clinical manifestations of syphilis. These include failure to thrive, skin rashes, hepatosplenomegaly, osteitis (which may lead to collapse of the bridge of the nose), epiphysitis, pneumonia due to an interstitial fibrosis, pericellular hepatic fibrosis, meningitis, choroidoretinitis, meningitis and anaemia. Later in life, iridocyclitis and periostitis (e.g.'sabre tibia') may develop. In adolescence, the child can develop interstitial keratitis leading to blindness, nerve deafness and optic nerve atrophy, gummas, general paralysis of the insane and tabes dorsalis. The teeth may show the typical Hutchinson's peg-shaped incisor and Moon's domed molars.

4. The placenta infected with treponemes is enlarged and pale, almost hydropic in appearance, and shows microscopical changes of endarteritis and fibrosis.

A 23-year-old singer of popular music, whom we shall call Ms J F, booked in her first pregnancy at 19 weeks gestation. She was currently resident in the United Kingdom, but had travelled extensively throughout Europe in the pursuit of her occupation. The putative father of the child was an Italian record producer, domiciled in Milan. Ms J F booked late because she had left Italy following a Christmas holiday in Milan without realising she was pregnant, and when the pregnancy had been confirmed at 9 weeks amenorrhoea she had returned to Milan to acquaint the putative father with the good news. Unfortunately, she found that he had been taken into hospital with pneumocystis carinii pneumonia. His human immunodeficiency virus (HIV) antibody titre was positive.

She was naturally devastated by this news and returned to the UK uncertain of what to do. She was frightened that she might have acquired HIV infection herself and had therefore been reluctant to present herself for medical care because it meant facing the implications of the condition for her future and, in particular, for her pregnancy.

During the booking interview, she wished to know whether she should be tested for carriage of the HIV virus, what the implications of the test (and in particular a positive result) would be for her life-style, what effect the infection would have on her pregnancy (and the effect of pregnancy on the disease), and the likely outcome for the child if she chose to continue with the pregnancy.

How would you answer these questions?

Testing for HIV infection is normally performed by detection of HIV antibody in the blood. A variety of tests can be used and most of them have a high sensitivity and specificity; results are usually double checked with several methods before reporting. This has reduced the risk of false positive reports to a very low level. Initially, antibody to the viral envelope proteins is assayed, but later in the course of the infection core protein antibodies also appear. In the late stages, antibody may disappear, overwhelmed by the load of antigen in the blood, but then HIV virus can be detected directly in the blood using tissue culture. The main difficulty with testing is the latent period between infection and the appearance of antibody; this is usually about 3 months but varies between 1 month and 1 year. Unfortunately, the carrier is probably particularly infectious during this period. For this and other reasons, there is no place for HIV testing simply to 'protect staff', as the possibility of infection exists even from HIV antibody-negative women. Birth attendants are, therefore, well advised to take appropriate precautions to prevent infection at all times, not just in the presence of a known infected individual.

Thus the decision as to whether a pregnant woman should be tested is ultimately one for the individual concerned, not for her medical attendant. In order to make the best decision, she needs as much information as possible. Although at one time it was thought that pregnancy accelerated the progression of HIV infection to full-blown acquired immunodeficiency syndrome (AIDS), it is now clear that this is not true. It is now also evident that HIV infection per se (as opposed to AIDS) has no effect on pregnancy; in particular it does not cause congenital malformation, intrauterine growth retardation, preterm labour or mental deficiency. Thus the major medical factor to be considered is the possibility of giving birth to a child with congenital HIV infection, the risk of which is currently estimated at about 30%. Most of these infected children will develop AIDS within the first 10 years of life. Some women may regard this risk as a justification for termination of the pregnancy. Other potential advantages to knowing that one is HIV positive include the possibility of improving life expectancy by drug treatment, such as with 3'-azido thymidine (AZT, Zidovudine, Retrovir), and the ability to modify sexual practices to minimise the risk of infecting others (so-called 'safe sex' procedures). In addition, the small risk of transmitting the infection to the neonate via breast milk can be avoided by bottle feeding.

Unfortunately, there are also many negative aspects to knowing one is HIV infected. These need to be discussed carefully with the woman before she is tested. They include severe depression and sometimes difficulty with personal relationships. There is a great deal of uninformed prejudice against HIV-positive persons, and the person being tested should consider carefully whether she should tell anyone about this before the result is known; if she is positive, then careful decisions need to be made about who should be told. An HIV-positive person is usually unable to obtain life insurance or a mortgage for property purchase; her ability to pursue her occupation may also be affected.

Ms J F chose to be tested, but despite careful counselling refused to allow the result to be communicated to her or her birth attendants. She was accordingly treated as infected and precautions to prevent transmission of infection to staff were emphasised. However, when the baby was 3 months of age, it became ill with pneumonia and Ms J F admitted to having developed chronic diarrhoea. She then accepted the information that both she and her daughter were HIV positive and treatment with careful follow-up were commenced.

Obstetrics 48

A 23-year-old woman booked for hospital confinement in the 12th week of her first pregnancy. The pregnancy progressed uneventfully until the 34th week when her blood pressure rose to 155/95 mmHg, and she developed ++ proteinuria. She was admitted to hospital for assessment and bed-rest, but as her blood pressure and proteinuria settled, she was allowed home a week later. She defaulted on her next appointment, but was admitted as an emergency at 38 weeks gestation with severe abdominal pain and slight vaginal bleeding.

On arrival on the labour ward she was pale with a pulse rate of 100 beats/minute and a blood pressure of 130/80 mmHg. The uterine size was compatible with dates but it was hard and tender; the fetal heart could not be heard.

An intravenous line was inserted in her left antecubital fossa and a central venous pressure line inserted in her right antecubital fossa. Blood was sent for urgent crossmatching and estimation of clotting factors. A rapid infusion of plasma substitute and fresh frozen plasma was commenced. Ultrasound scan confirmed abruptio placentae with a major placental separation and no evidence of fetal heart activity. Vaginal examination revealed a cervix dilated to 6 cm with the fetal head below the spines. An indwelling catheter was inserted into her bladder and a decision was made to await spontaneous labour progress. Her condition remained stable for the next hour but then it was noticed that she was bleeding from the sites of both her intravenous lines, and from the venepuncture site where the blood sample had been drawn.

1. What would you expect the clotting screen to show?
2. How would you correct the coagulation failure?
3. How would you deliver this patient?

1. The presence of a disseminated intravascular coagulopathy (DIC) was confirmed by a low platelet count (34000/μl, normal in pregnancy >100000/μl), a partial thromboplastin time of 76 seconds (control 40), a reduced fibrinogen concentration (104 mg/dl, normal 300–600 mg/dl in late pregnancy) and a raised level of fibrin degradation products (156 μg/ml, normal <100 μg/ml).

2. The most important steps in correcting coagulation failure are to remove the cause and maintain the circulating blood volume. The first is achieved by delivering the fetus as quickly as possible, the second by transfusing blood or blood products such as fresh frozen plasma, fibrinogen and platelets. A central venous pressure line is essential to assess the rate and adequacy of volume replacement. If the coagulation disorder persists for longer than 12 hours despite the above measures, the use of heparin should be considered. This apparently paradoxical therapy prevents further intravascular coagulation and allows fibrinogen and platelet levels to rise, with an improvement of clotting in the extravascular compartment. The guidance of an expert haematologist should always be sought before such a drastic step is taken.

3. Since the fetus was already dead, it had been hoped that she would deliver vaginally. However, the onset of coagulopathy meant that urgent delivery was necessary and a caesarean section was performed. Despite the presence of blood in the myometrium ('Couvelaire uterus') the uterus contracted strongly once the fetus, placenta and 700 ml of clot was delivered, and the uterine bleeding was controlled rapidly once the lower segment was sutured. Eight units of blood, 6 of fresh frozen plasma and 4 bags of platelets later, the generalised bleeding subsided and clotting returned to normal over the next 36 hours.

Obstetrics 49

A 25-year-old teacher had an elective caesarean section at 38 weeks gestation because of clinical cephalopelvic disproportion. This was her second pregnancy, the first having ended in an emergency caesarean section after a long labour with minimal descent of the fetal head.

The second caesarean was uncomplicated and a healthy female infant was delivered. The placenta was removed manually and the uterine cavity noted to be empty before closing the incision.

While breast feeding about 48 hours after delivery, the patient had a substantial vaginal bleed, resulting in shock, which required a 4-unit blood transfusion. The uterus had been involuting normally up until this time and even after the bleed was firm and well contracted. A speculum examination was performed once her condition was stable and no abnormality was found. The bleeding settled spontaneously and, as the uterus continued to involute normally, she was allowed home on the seventh postoperative day.

She was readmitted as an emergency with a further heavy bleed 4 days later and once again required resuscitation and transfusion. The bleeding settled spontaneously and an ultrasound scan showed no evidence of retained products of conception within the uterine cavity. The woman was at no time pyrexial and routine high vaginal swabs showed the growth of commensal organisms only. She went home 2 days later only to be admitted again after 12 hours with yet another substantial bleed. Once again the uterus was well contracted and no cervical or vaginal bleeding was seen on speculum examination.

1. What is the likelihood of her persistent bleeds being due to a coagulopathy?
2. The next step is clearly an examination under anaesthetic, but what procedures would you wish the woman to give informed consent for?
3. No abnormality is found at EUA; blood continues to issue from the os which accepts a 14 Hegar dilator without difficulty. The blood clots normally. What now?

1. The likelihood of these bleeds being due to a coagulopathy is small. If there is a very large bleed due to any cause, a disturbance of normal coagulation may occur, but then there would be other signs present — bleeding would occur from drip sites and the blood issuing from the vagina would not clot. If the patient had had an inherited bleeding disorder then it would almost certainly have been known about, or become apparent, at the time of the first caesarean section.

2. The patient should be asked to consent to whatever procedures may transpire to be necessary to stop the bleeding. This will certainly include an evacuation of the uterus, but may also include hysterectomy if all else fails.

3. In the absence of any obvious cause for the bleeding, and if no retained products are found, management should be directed towards preventing further bleeding. This usually means either packing the uterus, or performing a hysterectomy. In this case the patient was very keen to preserve her uterus and so, when no retained products were found, the uterus was packed with 2 cm wide gauze soaked in proflavine emulsion. Cefuroxime, metronidazole and gentamicin were given intravenously because of the possibility that endometritis was the cause of the bleeding. The patient was sent to the ward for close observation until the pack was removed in theatre the next morning. There was only slight vaginal loss over the next few days, during which time intravenous administration of antibiotic was continued, and the patient was finally allowed home for the third time after four days, to complete a week's course of oral cefuroxime and metronidazole. She had no further bleeding until a normal menstrual period 2 months later; subsequent menses were also normal.

    If the woman is determined to keep her uterus in this situation, it may be possible to arrest continuing haemorrhage by ligation of the internal iliac arteries. This is usually a difficult procedure because oedema of the pelvic peritoneum makes identification of the pelvic structures difficult (this includes the ureter). A urologist or general surgeon specialising in pelvic surgery should therefore be available to provide assistance for such a procedure.

    Endometritis is a potent cause of haemorrhage in the puerperium and should always be treated vigorously with adequate doses of appropriate antibiotics (particularly those active against Gram negative and anaerobic organisms), if necessary given intravenously.

Obstetrics 50

A 22-year-old woman contacted her GP complaining of frequency of micturition. Over the previous four years she had presented on a number of occasions with similar complaints and each time a urinary tract infection had been proven on urine culture before treatment with the appropriate antibiotic had been given.

On this occasion, her GP decided that these recurrent urinary infections needed further investigation and therefore arranged for her to have an intravenous urogram (IVU). Because of shortages of staff in the local hospital X-ray department, the IVU was delayed, and by the time the patient attended she had not had a period for 10 weeks. When asked if she might be pregnant the woman replied that she thought it unlikely because she and her partner always used a sheath for contraception and anyway her periods were often irregular. The IVU was performed and found to be normal. Three weeks later the woman reattended her general practitioner complaining of recurrent nausea, which she attributed to the after-effects of the IVU. A pregnancy test was positive and she was referred the next day to her local antenatal clinic, where an ultrasound confirmed that she was indeed pregnant, with a crown–rump length of 41.5 cm, equivalent to 11 weeks gestational age.

1. What would you advise the woman regarding the likely effects of the IVU on the pregnancy?
2. What dosage of radiation is embryopathic?
3. What precautions should be taken before X-raying a woman in the reproductive age group?

This lady would have been about 8 weeks pregnant at the time of her IVU. Exposure to irradiation in the second month of pregnancy has been shown to cause malformation in specific organs in experimental animals and irradiation of the forebrain between 8 and 15 weeks may result in mental retardation. It has been estimated that, in relation to diagnostic use of X-rays in the human, the risk of inducing derangement of organogenesis or cancer is of the order of 1 case per 1000 for every 1 cGy of radiation, although some interference with brain growth may occur in 5 per 1000 cases for every 1 cGy. However, nearly all modern X-ray equipment will use less than 1 cGy for an IVU, and even a barium enema usually requires no more than 2 cGy. Bearing in mind that the background rate of significant congenital anomaly in all pregnancies is 20 per 1000, the extra risk from the X-irradiation is relatively insignificant.

Accordingly, the British Institute of Radiology agreed with other national authorities in 1974 that an exposure of less than 10 cGy should not be considered grounds for termination of pregnancy, though later work suggested that 5 cGy was the upper limit when the irradiation occurred in the 10th to 15th weeks.

More recently, it has become apparent there may be a risk from irradiation of the ovum during the 7 weeks before ovulation. The formation of the zona pellucida coincides with a change in the nuclear morphology of the oocyte, during which time the oocyte appears to be particularly sensitive to the effects of radiation. It has been suggested that a dose of 1 cGy at this time increases the risk of mutation causing genetic disease by approximately 50-fold, to about 2.5 cases per 1000. Thus, it seems that the old 10-day rule' whereby X-ray investigations were only carried out in the 10 days following menstruation, when it was thought unlikely that a woman was pregnant, is illogical. Indeed, in 1984 the International Commission on Radiological Protection withdrew its support from the rule, and suggested that no special precautions were needed within 4 weeks of the last period (the '28-day rule'). However, in view of the potential risk to the ovum, perhaps the safest advice at the present time is to advise that, unless a woman of childbearing ability can be absolutely certain that she is not pregnant, and will not become pregnant in the next 7 weeks, X-ray examination should only be performed if deemed to be essential by the radiologist or referring clinician. If there is doubt about pregnancy, then a blood beta-HCG measurement should be performed and if it is negative then the woman should be advised to use an effective method of contraception for at least 8 weeks following any radiological investigation. However, if conception occurs despite this advice, then the woman should be reassured that the risk is small enough as to be almost insignificant and termination of pregnancy is not warranted on medical grounds unless the level of radiation exceeds 5 cGy.

Gynaecology 1

A 34-year-old housewife, married to a 36-year-old police officer, came to the gynaecology clinic complaining of secondary infertility. She had started her reproductive career at the age of 22, with a 10-week miscarriage. One year later, she had become pregnant again and this pregnancy had ended with a caesarean section at term for a persistent transverse lie.

Over the next 5 years the couple used the 'safe period' for contraception as they were Roman Catholic. The wife continued to have a regular 28-day menstrual cycle, which she had had since the menarche at 14 years of age.

Six years before the clinic visit they decided to have another child. During this time they were both reasonably well, although increasingly anxious about her failure to conceive.

Twelve months before the clinic visit the husband had a brief episode of haematuria, but full investigations including an IVU revealed no abnormality of the urinary or genital system. A month later his wife ceased to menstruate. She had therefore had 11 months amenorrhoea when she came to the clinic.

On closer questioning, she admitted to an episode of galactorrhoea 9 months previously. She had also noticed increasing constipation, loss of energy, and general malaise. Her skin had become dry and her hair dull. Her weight was, however, normal and steady.

On examination there was no apparent abnormality of the genital tract and she was not pregnant.

1. What further questions would you like to ask relating to her medical history?
2. Which aspects of the physical examination other than that of the genital tract are particularly important in this case?
3. Predict the results of her Hb, WBC, FSH and prolactin estimations.
4. Which further biochemical investigation is indicated?
5. Outline your management.

1. Any serious systemic illness or endocrine disturbance can give rise to amenorrhoea, and a full medical history is therefore important in the investigation of secondary amenorrhoea. In the present case, the significant features are the dry hair and skin together with constipation and malaise. These suggest hypothyroidism. Subsequent questioning revealed that she hated cold weather, kept the house so hot that her husband complained and had also noticed that her voice had become increasingly croaky.

2. When there is any suggestion of hypothyroidism the neck and the tendon reflexes must be carefully examined. This patient had a soft diffuse, non-tender enlargement of her thyroid gland (a thyroid-shaped goitre). Her reflexes, particularly the ankle jerks, were slowed and had a greatly prolonged relaxation time.

3. Anaemia is common in hypothyroidism, but in mild cases the haemoglobin concentration may be normal. In the present case it was 12.3 g/dl, with a normal white count of 7800/mm^3. Her FSH level was normal at 6.4 u/l. Ovulatory failure in patients with hypothyroidism seems to be due to disordered regulation of gonadotrophin secretion. Their anovulatory cycles may be associated either with prolonged and irregular uterine bleeding (unopposed oestrogen effect) or amenorrhoea (lack of progestogen withdrawal bleeding).

    Thyroid failure is usually autoimmune in origin (antithyroid antibodies can often be demonstrated) and is associated with increased TSH release (from the pituitary), possibly due to increased sensitivity to TRH (thyrotropin-releasing hormone). TRH also stimulates the release of prolactin and in the present case the prolactin level was 1084 mu/l, approximately 50% above the upper limit of normal. This may account for the galactorrhoea reported by the patient. It does not, however, necessarily explain her amenorrhoea, since treatment with bromocriptine (a dopamine agonist which suppresses prolactin secretion) does not restore ovulation, and indeed may exacerbate the hypothyroidism.

4. Full investigation of thyroid status is clearly mandatory in this case, and is probably wise in any case of unexplained amenorrhoea. The values in this case were (Table 5):

	Normal range in pregnancy
Thyroxine 39 nmol/l	(70–206)
TSH > 28 mu/l	(1–3.5)

5. Oral thyroxine is used to correct thyroid deficiency. The starting dose is 0.05 mg daily and this can be increased to 0.2 mg daily if necessary. Evaluation of the correct dose is best performed by using serial thyroid function tests rather than relying on clinical measures, since the patient may feel better but still be slightly hypothyroid. When the patient is euthyroid, menstruation and fertility normally resume without additional treatment.

Gynaecology 2

Mrs PS came to gynaecology outpatients at the age of 31, requesting reversal of sterilisation. Six years previously, she had been happily married, with 3 children aged 3 years 6 months, 2 years, and 5 months. She had been advised against taking the oral contraceptive (combined pill) because of horrendous varicose veins and as the IUCD caused heavy and painful periods, she requested sterilisation. This was performed via the laparoscope, with a Hulka-Clemens clip being applied to each tube. Nine months later her marriage broke down and her husband left home. She commenced a new relationship three years later, and had been cohabiting with her new partner for three years when she presented requesting reversal of sterilisation. Her new partner had no children of his own.

1. Comment on the initial decision to sterilise this woman at the age of 25.
2. Outline five special provisos that should be put to any woman before sterilisation is performed.
3. If you agreed to perform the reversal in this case, what further information would you need?
4. What procedure would you employ and what results might you expect?

1. Most gynaecologists in the United Kingdom will willingly sterilise a woman who is happily married, aged more than 30, and with two normal children. Should these conditions not be fulfilled, it is usual to make sure that all types of reversible contraception have been tried (the progestogen-only pill might have been suitable in this case) and to defer a decision for at least six months while a social report is obtained (this will include interviewing the husband).

2. Careful attention should be paid to the following points when discussing sterilisation with a couple requesting the procedure.
   1. They should be fully aware that the procedure is potentially irreversible.
   2. They should be aware that an inevitable (though small) anaesthetic and operative risk is involved in the procedure.
   3. Any woman who is to have a laparoscopic sterilisation should be asked whether she wishes the surgeon to continue via a `minilaparotomy' if laparoscopic sterilisation proves to be technically impossible.
   4. She should be aware that there is a 1 in 200–500 risk of failure of the procedure (i.e. that she might become pregnant).
   5. The partner should also be seen and asked to sign the consent form, after the procedure has been fully explained (his signature is not legally necessary but is advisable).

3. Before attempting a reversal, one should check the original notes to ensure that the fallopian tubes were healthy, and that there are no unfavourable features (such as two clips, widely separated, on one tube). It is also wise to exclude the chance of subsequent damage by asking about sexually transmitted diseases and attacks of salpingitis. Ovulation is confirmed most simply using a luteal phase progesterone estimation. A semen analysis should also be obtained from the new male partner before proceeding with reversal.

4. Simple excision of the clips and reanastomosis with 6/0 prolene (with or without a nylon splint) is sufficient to give an 80% reversal success rate without microsurgery. Mrs PS conceived a normal intrauterine pregnancy four months following reversal of sterilisation using this technique.

Gynaecology 3

A 33-year-old housewife had been married to a wire solderer for 8 years and had been trying unsuccessfully to become pregnant during this time. A laparoscopy when she was 29 showed no abnormality. When she was 31 she suddenly developed a swollen, purple left arm and shoulder. This resolved without treatment, but a subsequent venogram showed blockage of the left axillary and subclavian vein, with collateral flow through intercostal veins IV and V. She was anticoagulated with heparin and then with warfarin, 1 mg daily. All was well until 9 months later when she noticed progressive abdominal swelling. Her periods stopped, and at first she thought she was pregnant, but pregnancy tests were repeatedly negative. Investigation revealed an ESR of 62 mm/h, Hb 11.3 g/dl, WBC 4000, plasma urea 6.6 mmol/l, with normal electrolytes and liver function tests. Her prothrombin time was 29 seconds (control 13 seconds). An IVP showed normal renal function, but evidence of ascites.

She was admitted to hospital for investigation. Blood glucose and serum amylase were normal. Nine litres of fluid were obtained by paracentesis. The fluid contained cells which were of the glandular type, with frequent mitoses, suggestive of malignancy.

1. Which factors in the history favour a malignant aetiology for this woman's illness?
2. Suggest a possible benign aetiology for the paracentesis findings.
3. What is the next investigation you would suggest?
4. Why did she develop amenorrhoea?

1. Unheralded venous thrombosis may be due to a number of medical conditions, including infection and polycythaemia; but if there is no obvious cause it can sometimes be a prodromal condition related to occult neoplastic change. The classical form is known as thrombophlebitis migrans, and the thrombosis recurs in various sites. In this case, the course of the disease may have been modified by the anticoagulant therapy. The high ESR and evidence of ascites makes a malignant condition very likely. The possibility of primary liver disease, or pancreatitis, is excluded by normal biochemistry.

2. Surprisingly, the presence of apparently malignant adenocarcinoma cells in the paracentesis fluid is not prima facie evidence of carcinoma; fluid from an ovarian cyst can contain cells shed from the cyst lining which exhibit features suggestive of malignancy if they are found free in peritoneal fluid. Benign ovarian cysts rank amongst the largest benign tumours which can occur, and for one to contain 9 litres of fluid is not extraordinary. It can be impossible clinically to differentiate between a large flaccid ovarian cyst and ascites; the appearance may also be indistinguishable radiologically, but can often be differentiated with an ultrasound scan. When apparently tapping ascites, it is always possible that one is actually aspirating fluid from an ovarian cyst.

3. The only diagnostic procedure in this situation is laparotomy, and this was performed in the present case. Bilateral, friable ovarian cysts were found, with secondaries on the anterior wall of the uterus, rendering the bladder completely adherent. There was no evidence of secondaries elsewhere in the abdomen. Both ovaries were removed, as was the omentum, but hysterectomy was not performed to avoid damage to the bladder. Histology confirmed a well-differentiated papillary cystadenoma with some foci of malignant change, and the presence of psammoma bodies.

4. Amenorrhoea is a common, non-specific response to any severe and debilitating illness and this was probably the cause in this case.

   Following further evaluation with CAT scanning and ultrasound, and detailed renal function tests, she was treated with 8 MeV radiotherapy, 24 treatments over 53 days. Total tumour dose was 2340 rad, and the total pelvic dose 4340 rad. Follow-up therapy was with chlorambucil 10 mg daily for 6 weeks, repeated at 3-monthly intervals provided her white count was greater than $2500/mm^3$, and platelets more than $100000/mm^3$.

   She remained well two years after operation.

Gynaecology 4

A 55-year-old unmarried library assistant visited her GP complaining of generalised muscular aches, weakness and a slight cough. General examination revealed no abnormality, but investigation revealed an ESR of 75 mm/hour. Over the next three months many investigations were carried out, including blood urea and electrolyte estimation; the mono-spot test (for glandular fever), liver function tests, complement fixation tests for seven virus infections, latex factor estimation; thyroid antibody titre, thyroid function tests, testing for occult blood in the stool, sputum cytology, urine culture, cervical smear cytology, barium meal and follow through. All these investigations were normal. It was, however, discovered that she had a marked increase in plasma alpha-1 and alpha-2 globulins, and a marked diffuse increase in plasma gamma globulins. No myeloma band was seen.

She then began to lose weight and was referred to outpatients. At this time, she was found to have a normal chest X-ray, a haemoglobin of 10.5 g/dl with a normal serum iron and total iron binding capacity, a negative Brucella complement fixation test, a negative antinuclear factor screen and no DNA antibodies. Blood glucose and serum amylase were also normal. The plasma protein abnormalities were confirmed. Ascites was diagnosed clinically, and gynaecological examination showed a firm mass in the pelvis the size of a 10-week pregnancy. Paracentesis showed adenoma cells with appearances suggestive of malignancy. An intravenous urogram was normal. Ultrasound scanning confirmed the presence of an abdominal mass but the pelvic organs appeared normal.

A laparotomy was performed via a lower midline incision, which revealed a large tumour mass in the omentum. There was no evidence of tumour elsewhere; the liver, uterus and ovaries all appeared normal. Seven litres of ascitic fluid were removed.

1. What operative procedure would you perform?
2. How would you close the abdomen?
3. If the histology confirmed adenocarcinoma, suggest appropriate follow-up therapy.

1. It is a fundamental principle of most cancer surgery that as much malignant tissue as possible be removed surgically before adjuvant treatment is attempted. This is known as 'debulking'. In this case, the whole omentum was removed. It was then necessary to decide whether the uterus and ovaries should be removed. The commonest sites of adenocarcinoma in the abdomen are the stomach, pancreas and ovaries. In this case there was no evidence of a gastric or pancreatic lesion; occult primary carcinoma in the ovaries can lead to widespread secondary deposits elsewhere in the abdomen. There is nothing to favour conservation of the uterus and ovaries in a postmenopausal woman, other than the slight increase in operative risk, and total hysterectomy and bilateral salpingo-oophorectomy was therefore performed.

2. The danger in any debilitated person following a major abdominal operation is dehiscence of the wound. This is particularly likely where there is a possibility of recurrent ascites. Many surgeons now favour 'mass closure' of the wound with interrupted nylon sutures, including all layers of the abdomen except skin (which is closed separately). This type of closure is associated with a very low rate of dehiscence. Some surgeons might also favour a corrugated rubber — or tube — drain, 3 cm lateral to the wound, to ensure that ascites does not accumulate in the immediate postoperative period.

3. The histology confirmed poorly differentiated adenocarcinoma, with foci in the ovaries suggesting that they were indeed the primary source of the neoplasm.
   Follow-up therapy in this type of case would be with a cytotoxic agent such as cisplatin intravenously every 3 weeks for 6–9 months. This was, in fact, given to the patient described following a good recovery from her operation. An audiogram and renal function tests were normal (cisplatin is both oto- and nephrotoxic). She was preloaded with 2 litres of normal saline plus 1 g KC1 given intravenously over 12 hours to protect her kidneys by producing a diuresis, and then infused with 100 mg of cisplatin intravenously. This was 'covered' with metoclopramide and promethazine because this drug usually induces severe nausea and vomiting. A further 2 litres of normal saline and KC1 were given over the subsequent 12 hours. She was given 5 courses of 100 mg of cisplatin at 3-weekly intervals, then 5 further doses of 50 mg. She was alive and well 2 years after commencing therapy. Audiograms and renal function tests preceding each treatment showed some deterioration (high frequency hearing loss, and a drop in creatinine clearance from 100 to 60 ml per minute) suggesting that a further course of therapy with this agent would not be advisable; signs of recurrence would be treated with chlorambucil.

Gynaecology 5

A 34-year-old hairdresser was referred from the 'special clinic' for sexually transmitted disease because of an acute exacerbation of chronic lower abdominal pain.

She had one daughter aged 16; 8 years previously a right tubal ectopic pregnancy had been removed by right salpingectomy. Her appendix had been removed before the birth of her first child. She had attended the special clinic 12 months previously and a diagnosis of gonorrhoea had been made, for which she had received a full course of therapy. Her boyfriend had also been treated; he was her regular sexual partner and the couple never used any contraception as they wished to have a child. She continued to have some lower abdominal pain and a diagnosis of chronic salpingitis was made. She received three courses of antibiotics over the next year, with some relief of symptoms each time.

On the day she presented, she gave a 2-day history of increasing pain in the right iliac fossa. It was constant, worse on deep breathing, and made her nauseated. Her last menstrual period had been 15 days previously and was normal; her cycle was regular, 5/27. She had noticed a brown vaginal loss for 48 hours and she had passed either a clot of blood or some 'tissue'.

On examination, she was apyrexial, and vital signs were normal (pulse 80 beats/minute, blood pressure 120/80). She was tender with marked guarding and 'rebound' tenderness in the right iliac fossa. Vaginal examination did not reveal any bleeding and the cervix was closed and firm. A large mass was palpable on the right side of the uterus, which was extremely tender; a smaller, non-tender mass was also present on the left side. The uterus itself was not enlarged.

1. Discuss the features favouring or against:
   (i)   a further ectopic pregnancy
   (ii) an acute exacerbation of pelvic inflammatory disease
   (iii) an ovarian cyst.
2. What further investigations would you suggest before proceeding to laparotomy?
3. Discuss your management should she have:
   (i)   a further ectopic pregnancy
   (ii) a 10 cm diameter hydrosalpinx
   (iii) a 10 cm diameter ovarian cyst.

1. (i)   A potent predisposing factor to ectopic pregnancy is damage to the fallopian tube, such as can be caused by pelvic inflammatory disease. A diagnosis of ectopic pregnancy must, therefore, always be considered when a woman with a history of pelvic inflammation, or a previous ectopic, presents with lower abdominal pain. However, in this case, the apparently normal menstrual period 15 days previously is against such a diagnosis (although the possibility still exists that it was abnormal bleeding rather than a true period). In addition, the pain was on the right and the right tube had been removed (although it should be remembered that ectopic pregnancy can occur in the remaining stump of tube following salpingectomy).
    (ii)   Pelvic inflammatory disease tends to become chronic and a recurrence must always be considered when an affected patient presents with lower abdominal pain; however, in this case the lack of pyrexia is against the diagnosis (although it would be important to check that her temperature had not been suppressed with antibiotics). The pelvic masses are potentially inflammatory in origin, but the unilateral tenderness is unusual, especially as it is maximal on the side of her salpingectomy.
    (iii)   In any patient presenting with acute lower abdominal pain but no temperature, an accident to an ovarian cyst should be considered.
2. Tenderness often precludes a definitive pelvic examination, and laparoscopy is usually the investigation of choice in order to decide whether a laparotomy is necessary. Haemoglobin estimation, blood grouping and saving of serum are necessary before operation.
3. (i)   A further ectopic pregnancy would have to be removed; the main problem would be whether any attempt at tubal conservation is practical if the patient wishes to preserve fertility. This has to be discussed fully with the patient before operation, and the risk of further ectopics explained should she opt for tubal conservation.
    (ii)   Hydrosalpinges should not normally be removed if found incidentally, as this may cause a severe exacerbation of pelvic inflammation. The commonest indication for removal is torsion, leading to necrosis and abdominal pain. Recurrent infection is best treated with antibiotics unless a very large pyosalpinx is found.
    (iii)   An ovarian cyst 10 cm or more in diameter should always be removed surgically; if there is any doubt whether it is malignant (e.g. the presence of solid areas) the entire ovary is best removed with every attempt to avoid rupture. At the age of 34, especially if further fertility is required, it is not usual to remove the other ovary, the uterus and the omentum, unless there is clear evidence (such as the presence of secondary deposits) of malignancy. Further procedures depend on the pathology report on the cyst.
    In the case described, a 10 cm ovarian cyst of the right ovary was found. The right ovary was removed, complete with cyst. Histology showed it to be an endodermal sinus tumour, a very malignant tumour originating in primitive pluripotent ovarian cells. It had been completely removed and had not penetrated the wall of the cyst. No further operative procedure was performed, but she

was followed up with the use of the tumour markers carcinoembryonic antigen (CEA), alpha-fetoprotein (AFP) and beta-HCG, with a view to chemotherapy if there were signs of recurrence.

Other important investigations in this situation are (blood) urea and electrolytes, liver function tests, a chest X-ray, intravenous urography, and computerised axial tomography of the abdomen (to detect involved lymph nodes).

Gynaecology 6

A 24-year-old Italian nun, unable to speak English, presented in casualty one evening at 11 p.m. Through an interpreter, it was established that she had been completely well until the early afternoon, when she developed mild lower abdominal pain. This became more severe as the day progressed, and she began to vomit undigested food at about 9 p.m. The pain had commenced centrally, about 2 cm below the umbilicus, and had then spread to the right iliac fossa. There were no urinary symptoms, and she had previously been in good health.

On examination, she was obviously distressed, but vital signs were normal (pulse 76/minute, blood pressure 130/90). She was afebrile.

Abdominal examination revealed marked tenderness in the right iliac fossa. Vaginal examination confirmed that she was virgo intacta, but with one finger it was possible to feel the cervix only 5 cm from the introitus.

Her haemoglobin was 13.0 g/dl, with a white count of 11 400/mm^3. Urea and electrolytes were normal.

1. What part of the physical examination has been omitted?
2. Why is the cervix so easily palpable?
3. What is the likely diagnosis?

1. When a woman is virgo intacta, an adequate vaginal examination may be difficult, particularly if tampons are not used regularly. If so, a rectal examination should always be performed. In the case described, rectal examination clearly revealed the presence of a smooth mass, approximately 8 cm in diameter filling the pouch of Douglas.

2. The cervix was easily palpable because of the presence of the pelvic mass pushing the uterus down. A large uterine tumour could have the same effect.

3. The most likely diagnosis in a woman of this age is an incident involving an ovarian cyst, either torsion or bleeding into the cyst, or both. Rupture, with intra-abdominal bleeding, is unlikely in view of the normal vital signs. A less likely diagnosis is degeneration of a large fibroid; this would be unusual at the age of 24.

    Laparotomy confirmed an apparently benign 8 cm ovarian cyst, twisted three times on its pedicle. It was removed complete (including all the necrotic tissue — ovary and tube). Histology showed it to be a benign dermoid cyst.

Gynaecology 7

A 39-year-old school worker was referred to the gynaecology outpatients with a request for sterilisation. She had 3 children, aged 14, 8 and 7 years, all born normally at term. She had had no miscarriages or terminations of pregnancy.

Following her last pregnancy, she had used the combined oral contraceptive pill for 4 years, but it was discontinued when she complained of headaches, and her general practitioner found her blood pressure to be raised. She then had an intrauterine contraceptive device inserted.

Three months prior to her visit to outpatients , she had noticed some swelling of her breasts, which became tender, and she also had intermittent nausea. Her period, which was a few days later than her normal 29 days cycle, was very heavy and prolonged, and she developed aching lower abdominal pain in both groins. Her GP treated her with ampicillin, 500 mg qds for 10 days, with little improvement in the groin pain, although the breast tenderness and nausea subsided. She continued to have intermittent mild vaginal bleeding for the next three months.

When seen in the clinic, she still had some lower abdominal discomfort and a moderate reddish-brown vaginal loss. She was happily married and her husband supported her request for sterilisation. The risks of complications, failure rate, and irreversibility, were fully explained to, and accepted by, the patient. A urine latex agglutination pregnancy test was negative.

On examination, she was slightly tender in the suprapubic region, but there was no rebound or guarding. The uterus was retroverted and rather tender but was not obviously enlarged. There were no palpable adnexal masses. The coil was removed and she was given a prescription for co-trimoxazole, two tablets twice daily, and metronidazole, 200 mg three times daily.

1. What investigations were organised prior to her admission?
2. When would you admit her for sterilisation?
3. What technique of sterilisation would you recommend in this case?
4. Describe the consent form you would ask her to sign.
5. Why has she got prolonged vaginal bleeding?

1. The tests which were carried out were related firstly to the proposed sterilisation; these were a haemoglobin estimation, blood grouping and cervical smear; and secondly to her complaint of abdominal pain. These tests were cervical, urethral and rectal swabs placed in Stewart's transport medium, with instructions to culture for the gonococcus; a midstream urine specimen sent for microscopy, culture and sensitivity; an erythrocyte sedimentation rate (ESR); white blood cell count; a serum beta-HCG estimation, and a pelvic ultrasound scan.

   Her Hb was 9.6 g/dl, blood group ARh+ve. White count was 14 000/mm^3. The ESR was 46 mm/hour. Urine microscopy was normal and culture showed no growth. Culture of the swabs showed trichomonas vaginalis, as did the smear which showed no evidence of malignancy. The serum beta-HCG was reported as showing a level of 50 iu per litre. The ultrasound scan showed no evidence of any intrauterine gestation, but a diffuse echogenicity in the region of the left ovary, which could not be visualized clearly.

2. This lady has had abnormal vaginal bleeding for three months and should therefore be admitted as a matter of some urgency to establish the cause of her bleeding; she was admitted six days later for diagnostic curettage and laparoscopy. In addition, the low level of beta-HCG present suggests the possibility of a chronic ectopic pregnancy, a recent early miscarriage, or a very early intrauterine pregnancy.

3. It was intended to sterilise her by occluding her fallopian tubes with either the Hulka-Clemens clip or the Falope ring via the laparoscope, as this minimises inpatient stay, but in view of the possibility of complications making the procedure difficult via the laparoscope, the use of 'mini-laparotomy' was entertained.

4. This was fully explained to the patient so that she signed not only the usual consent form for sterilisation acknowledging irreversibility, but also consented specifically to a laparotomy if necessary and possible salpingectomy. She also consented to a D & C to exclude retained products of conception and the possibility of a very early intrauterine gestation (which she did not wish to continue). It was also considered possible that she might have had sepsis secondary to the coil and that this might make tubal visualisation difficult. In addition, some workers have suggested that use of clips or rings can exacerbate pelvic sepsis and that a Pomeroy procedure, with use of pelvic drain and antibiotic therapy, is preferable if sepsis is encountered at the time of sterilisation.

5. Chronic endometritis secondary to the coil can certainly cause prolonged uterine bleeding, but the breast tenderness and nausea in this case suggested the possibility of incomplete abortion or ectopic pregnancy, a suspicion strengthened by the low level of beta-HCG in the blood (at a level insufficient to show up in the standard latex agglutination urine pregnancy test). Dysfunctional uterine bleeding (due to hormonal disturbance) was thought to be unlikely.

   In the event, laparoscopy revealed a chronic left tubal ectopic pregnancy. The soft, necrotic tissue could not be palpated bimanually and the mass was walled off by flimsy adhesions. A left salpingectomy was performed via a Pfannenstiel incision, with removal of a small segment of right tube. Histology confirmed organising thrombus within the left fallopian tube, containing degenerating chorionic villi.

Gynaecology 8

A 24-year-old solicitor attended the gynaecology clinic worried because she had had only 2 very light periods in the previous 5 months. Her menarche had occurred when she was 11 years old and for the next 8 years she bled for 3 days every 4–6 weeks, following which the duration of her flow increased to 5 days every month. She was single, had never been pregnant, but had become sexually active 2 years prior to presentation. She had a coil inserted at the beginning of the relationship and had it removed again when the relationship ended after 18 months. She had had no further intercourse before she came to the clinic.

She had no other gynaecological symptoms. She had no headaches or galactorrhoea, but had used 'Colofac' for constipation about once a week for the previous year. She liked hot weather and had noticed her voice deepening recently. Her hair had become dry and coarse. She said she liked her work and had put in even more effort since her relationship had ended; she worried a lot and had lost about 4 kg in weight in the previous 9 months. She also felt rather tired and listless.

On examination she was 173 cm tall and weighed 54 kg. Her breasts, hair and thyroid appeared normal. Abdominal examination was normal. Vaginal examination showed a dry vagina with reddened, smooth epithelium. Her uterus was very small and anteverted. There were no adnexal masses.

Laboratory investigations showed the following results (normal range in parentheses): prolactin 106 mu/l (<360), thyroxine 96 nmol/l (70–160), random TSH <1 mu/l (1–3.5), FSH 7.0 u/l (1–10), LH 4.2 u/l (<14) and testosterone 2.5 nmol/l. A cervical smear was normal.

1. Why has she got oligomenorrhoea?
2. Give an explanation for the voice and hair changes and the constipation despite normal thyroid function tests.
3. What treatment would you recommend?

1. The most likely explanation for this woman's oligomenorrhoea is that she is underweight. Her body mass index (weight in kg divided by height in metres squared — normal range 19–25) was only 18. Even for a 'small frame' woman, the minimum normal body weight is 56 kg for someone 173 cm tall. When a woman's weight is at the lower limit of normal, the loss of as little as 4 kg can produce cessation of menstruation. The exact mechanism of this effect is not certain, but may be partly related to reduced oestrogen production from the diminished adipose tissue mass. Certainly this woman's atrophic vagina provided evidence suggestive of reduced oestrogenisation. However, the hypothalamus must also be involved in weight-related amenorrhoea, since despite the abnormally low oestrogen levels, gonadotrophin levels are not elevated.

2. Excessive weight loss is often an abnormal response to stress, particularly that related to adolescence and to personal relationships, as in this case. Indeed, it may progress in some cases to an overt psychiatric disorder, anorexia nervosa. Amenorrhoea may also be related to other emotional disturbances, such as depression. Depression produces symptoms such as retarded affect, tiredness and early morning waking. Somatic signs, such as dry skin and hair, husky voice and constipation, are also common.

3. In the present case, laboratory test results show that physical therapy was not indicated. The probable cause of the amenorrhoea, low body weight, was explained to the patient, who was rather sceptical. This is a common reaction, since many of these women appear to have an abnormal body image of themselves and think they are normal, although they are strikingly thin to observers. In view of the symptoms suggestive of depression, a psychiatric assessment was recommended but refused. The patient declined to attend for a further appointment, so a full report was sent to the general practitioner. This emphasised the need for psychiatric referral should the patient present with more serious symptoms or signs in the future. Early commencement of psychiatric treatment would be important in the prevention of the serious complication of anorexia nervosa, which may be fatal. However, most cases of weight-related amenorrhoea pursue a benign, intermittently relapsing course.

Gynaecology 9

Nine weeks after she married for the first time, a 35-year-old secretary attended the clinic worried that her amenorrhoea for the previous 4 years would prevent her conceiving. Her menarche had occurred at the age of 12, but her periods had always been infrequent with bleeding for 5–6 days every 9–12 weeks. At the age of 30 she had commenced regular sexual intercourse with the partner she eventually married. For the first 6 months, she used the combined oral contraceptive pill, but stopped because of excessive weight gain. Following this, her partner used sheaths. She had always been generally well, with no psychiatric problems. Her sense of smell was normal and she was not taking any medication. She had never had tuberculosis, appendicitis, or venereal disease. Her 30-year-old husband was also healthy and sexual intercourse was frequent and normal.

On examination, Mrs H was 166 cm tall and weighed 68 kg. She had normal female secondary sexual characteristics, with a female escutcheon. Vaginal and pelvic examination was also normal. Her visual fields were tested to confrontation and there was a suggestion of a small left temporal defect.

Further investigation was organised and she was given medroxy-progesterone acetate 5 mg t.d.s for 5 days, with instructions to take clomiphene 50 mg daily for 5 days if she had a withdrawal bleed following the provera. A plasma progesterone estimation was arranged for 12 days after finishing the clomiphene, if taken.

1. Which additional symptom would you have liked to ask about?
2. Which blood tests were organised, in addition to the progesterone?
3. What additional investigations are indicated in this case, and why?
4. Did she have a withdrawal bleed following the progesterone?
5. Suggest the cause of her amenorrhoea.

1. With prolonged secondary amenorrhoea as in this case 20% of women are eventually found to have hyperprolactinaemia. Half of these women will have galactorrhoea and this symptom should always be elicited by direct questioning (although galactorrhoea may occur in women with normal prolactin levels). This patient did not have galactorrhoea.

2. All women with secondary amenorrhoea (greater than 4 months) should have a haemoglobin and white blood count estimation (normal in this case), an FSH measurement (7 u/l, excluding ovarian failure), and thyroid function tests (thyroxine 94 nmol/l and TSH 3.2 mu/l, excluding thyroid dysfunction). Her prolactin was >4000 mu/l, indicating very marked hyperprolactinaemia. This was already suspected because of the visual field defect, which resulted from a pituitary adenoma compressing the optic chiasma.

3. This symptom meant that, at the initial visit, formal optometric visual field testing was arranged, as was a lateral skull X-ray with tomograms of the pituitary fossa (CAT scans are best organised by the endocrinologist, or neurosurgeon, if the patient proves to have a tumour). In cases without symptoms or signs of hyperprolactinaemia, it is sufficient to await the result of the serum prolactin estimation; these additional investigations are unnecessary if the prolactin value is normal.

4. This woman had no symptoms or signs of oestrogen deficiency and the progestogen withdrawal test was positive, indicating that progesterone receptors had been induced in the endometrium by circulating oestrogen. Clomiphene did not, however, produce ovulation. This is usual in cases of hyperprolactinaemia as the gonadotrophin response is deficient.

5. The 'catch' in this case is to label Mrs H as having post-pill amenorrhoea. This is a description, not a diagnosis and, although a woman who stops oral contraception is more likely to have clomiphene responsive (i.e. hypothalamic) amenorrhoea, especially if she gives a history of oligo- or amenorrhoea before using the pill, she is just as likely to have an organic lesion such as a pituitary adenoma and polycystic ovaries, or a psychiatric disorder such as anorexia nervosa, as a woman who has never taken the combined pill. All such cases must therefore be fully investigated, as above.

    Mrs H's skull X-rays showed a double floor to the pituitary fossa. A pituitary adenoma was confirmed by CAT scanning and an air encephalogram. She was treated with external irradiation and bromocriptine, whereupon she developed ovulatory menstrual cycles.

Gynaecology 10

A 27-year-old Ugandan Asian bank clerk had left Africa 6 years previously. Now married for 4 years, she presented to the clinic anxious because she had not conceived after 6 months without contraception. Her menarche had been at the age of 14 and since that time her periods had always been irregular, every 21–25 days, until she commenced the pill when she married. She was originally on Microgynon 30 but changed to Eugynon 30 because of breakthrough bleeding; on Eugynon 30 she had normal, regular withdrawal bleeds. She had stopped the pill on 30 June, had no period in July and then had periods commencing on 5 August, 19 September and 10 November; these periods had lasted from 3–5 days and had been scanty in amount.

She had no history of dyspareunia or intermenstrual bleeding, nor any other gynaecological symptoms. She had been very thin before marriage but had put on weight since and weighed 53 kg (she was 1.61 m tall). A chest X-ray had been normal on her arrival in the UK, and she had never had salpingitis or a sexually transmitted disease. She had never had a blood transfusion and her husband had been her only sexual partner. She did not have any galactorrhoea and suffered occasional 'tension' type headaches. Her hair and skin were healthy and she tolerated cold weather normally.

On examination she appeared to be a normal healthy female. She had well developed breasts with some hairiness around the areolae and a male-type escutcheon. Her vulva, vagina and cervix were normal and the uterus was small, anteverted and mobile. Both ovaries were palpable, slightly tender and about 7 cm in diameter.

1. Describe the expected hormone profile of this woman.
2. What pathological condition do you think she has?
3. What other investigations would you recommend?
4. Describe the treatment you would employ.

1. A plasma testosterone of 3.7 nmol/l (normal, 1–3 nmol/l) confirmed the clinical diagnosis of 'polycystic ovary' syndrome. Her LH concentration was elevated to 19.5 u/l, which is also typical; a plasma progesterone of less than 3.2 nmol/l 10 days after the LH measurement made it unlikely that this was due to a midcycle LH surge, since ovulation had clearly not occurred. The FSH concentration was normal (7.2 u/l). Thyroxine was 119 nmol/l (normal 70–160) and TSH 3.2 u/l (normal 1–3.5), confirming that she was euthyroid.

2. In polycystic ovarian disease (PCO) there is an excess of androgen which interferes with normal menstrual cycling by its action on the hypothalamus. The excess androgen is thought to come from the ovary and, to a lesser extent, from the adrenals. PCO was originally described in obese, hirsute women as the Stein-Leventhal syndrome, but essentially the same pathology can occur in slim women, as in this case.

3. The hormonal diagnosis can be confirmed using high resolution ultrasound; an abdominal transducer is usually sufficient, but in obese women use of a vaginal probe is often necessary to give a clear picture of the ovaries. The ultrasound appearance is characteristic; an ovary enlarged by 50-100% and with a string of follicles 1–2 cm in diameter surrounding the central stroma. It should be noted, however, that these appearances can be found in 15% of the total female population in the reproductive age group, many of whom will have no reproductive dysfunction. The ultrasound findings should, therefore, always be taken in conjunction with the clinical presentation and the hormonal profile. Confirmation by laparoscopy of the typically thickened, glistening white capsules of the enlarged, cystic ovaries is traditional, but not nowadays necessary either for diagnostic or therapeutic purposes.

4. The primary complaint of the patient may be unwanted hair, or, as in this case, infertility. Once the husband's sperm count was shown to be normal, she was treated with clomiphene to induce ovulation. She did not conceive with 50 mg on days 2–7 of the cycle, but increasing the dose to 100 mg per day produced a progesterone level of 55 nmol/l 2 weeks later. She conceived following the next course and subsequently gave birth to a healthy female weighing 2.82 kg. If clomiphene alone is unsuccessful, intramuscular injection of 10000 iu of HCG on day 10 may produce ovulation. Pergonal therapy is occasionally necessary; the success rate of this therapy may be improved by prior suppression of the hypothalamo-ovarian axis with long-acting GNRH analogue (buserelin). Pulsatile subcutaneous infusion of pure FSH (Metrodin) may be more successful than Pergonal in some women. Wedge resection of the ovaries (which probably acts by reducing androgen levels due to loss of ovarian tissue) is a 'traditional' treatment now used only as a last resort.
    If hirsuties is a problem, cyproterone acetate (an antiandrogen), plus ethinyl oestradiol (to suppress the ovaries) is often helpful. Dexamethasone (to suppress the adrenals) has also been used.

Gynaecology 11

A 27-year-old clerk worked for a recorded music company. She was married and had 2 children, aged 9 and 7. Both had been born normally at term. One year after the birth of her second child, she had become pregnant again. She felt she would not cope with a third child by the age of 21 and a therapeutic termination of pregnancy was requested and performed. At the same time a laparoscopic sterilisation was performed using diathermy.

The following year she had acute appendicitis and the 'offending organ' was removed surgically. At the age of 24, she developed lower abdominal pain and was admitted to hospital, where a laparoscopy was performed. A diagnosis of pelvic inflammatory disease was made and she was treated with antibiotics. She made a good recovery, but three months before the current presentation she experienced a recurrence of the symptoms. The pain became severe, especially in the groins and suprapubically. She felt generally unwell and her normally regular periods became irregular with bleeding at intervals of 9–15 days. Her family doctor treated her with antibiotics and progestagens, but the bleeding became worse. She also experienced intermittent dyspareunia.

On the day of admission she suffered a severe exacerbation of her pain, which she could time precisely to 16.15 hours. She did not vomit, but felt sick. She felt faint and had pain at the tips of both shoulders.

On examination she was acutely distressed and restless, but afebrile. She was tender in the right iliac fossa and vaginal examination revealed no uterine bleeding but marked cervical excitation and tenderness in the right fornix. The uterus was slightly enlarged, anteverted and mobile.

1. What is the significance of the shoulder tip pain; and how would you relate it to the feeling of faintness?
2. What is the most important haematological procedure which should be carried out?
3. List the differential diagnosis.

1. Shoulder tip pain is often referred pain from the diaphragm. The commonest gynaecological cause is blood in the peritoneal cavity, which tracks up the paracolic gutters and irritates the undersurface of the diaphragm. This, coupled with a feeling of faintness, should suggest the possibility of significant intraperitoneal bleeding with hypotension. This leads to a reduction of cerebral perfusion with consequent restlessness, as illustrated in this case. Ultimately, further signs of shock will appear, such as cold, pale skin (peripheral circulatory failure) and sweating (adrenergic response) with a tachycardia (an attempt to maintain cardiac output).

2. In this situation, the most vital procedure is to instigate the cross-matching of at least four units of blood, with a warning to the haematologist that more might be required; in an otherwise healthy young person, at least two units of blood need to be lost before obvious signs of shock appear.

3. The most likely diagnoses are haemorrhage into an ovarian cyst, with or without rupture, and ectopic pregnancy. Sterilisation does not rule out this latter diagnosis since recanalisation of the fallopian tubes can occur (this is an important cause of failure of laparoscopic sterilisation). Laparoscopy in this case showed a large amount of free blood in the peritoneal cavity and at laparotomy a ruptured right ampullary ectopic pregnancy was found. A three-unit blood transfusion was necessary to restore blood volume. Following removal of the ectopic pregnancy, the patient made an uneventful recovery.

Gynaecology 12

A 37-year-old housewife presented to the clinic complaining of persistent right iliac fossa pain since her sterilisation 6 months previously. She was married to a printer's assistant aged 40 and had two children aged 14 and 11. She had been made redundant from her job as canteen assistant 2 months before.

Ten years previously she had had severe marital difficulties and was admitted to a psychiatric hospital for 2 weeks. She was then well for 4 years, when she suddenly developed acute retention of urine. She had 5 urethral dilatations at 3-monthly intervals before her problem resolved.

She had used the coil for contraception since her last child, but developed dyspareunia which she attributed to the device. She therefore requested sterilisation and removal of the coil. She was sterilised by bilateral application of Hulka-Clemens clips. At the time of laparoscopy, her pelvis was noted to be normal, except for a 1 cm size ovarian cyst in the right ovary.

Since the sterilisation her dyspareunia had worsened and she also developed symptoms of tiredness, light headedness and painful breasts.

On examination she had a normal-sized anteverted mobile uterus with no excitation pain or tenderness. The left adnexum was entirely normal. The right ovary was slightly enlarged (about 3 cm diameter) and there was some tenderness when it was squeezed. She had not had intercourse for 3 months. She visited the outpatient clinic where a blood sample revealed a haemoglobin of 13.6 g/dl, a white count of 6500/mm^3 and an ESR of 2 mm/hour. An ultrasound examination confirmed the presence of a small right ovarian cyst.

1. Discuss the aetiology of her pain.
2. What further investigations are indicated?
3. Outline a plan of management.

1. This woman presents a typical example of the so-called 'pelvic pain syndrome'. The diagnosis rests on three main elements. Firstly, there is a history of psychiatric disturbance related to her sexual partner. The initial manifestation of this was overt, with psychiatric treatment necessary. The second was occult, the sudden onset of acute urinary retention. This is rare in women and in a high proportion has a hysterical origin. The absence of an organic cause, such as a tumour involving the urethra or neurological dysfunction (of which the commonest is disseminated sclerosis), is attested to by the repeated urethral dilatations without further investigations or treatment. Her sudden recovery was unlikely to be related to this procedure. Dyspareunia is also a common feature and may be either deep or superficial (due to vaginismus or excessive vaginal hygiene, e.g douching or deodorants causing vaginitis). Secondly, following a precipitating event (in this case, sterilisation; but it may be an attack of salpingitis, a miscarriage, or similar crisis) she developed a whole range of unrelated, occasionally bizarre, symptoms. Lightheadedness and tiredness are common manifestations of anxiety. Thirdly, physical examinations and investigations were all normal. Cystic enlargement of the ovary which does not exceed 4 cm in diameter can be considered within normal limits and all ovaries are slightly tender when subjected to bimanual compression.

2. With a normal haemoglobin, an ESR of 2 mm/hour and a recent normal laparoscopy, further investigations are not indicated and may only serve to confirm the patient in her belief that her symptoms must have an organic basis.

3. The main hope in therapy is to enable her to develop some insight and accept that her problems have an emotional basis. Counselling from a psychosexual expert or a marriage guidance counsellor is often helpful. An improvement in the patient's relationship frequently leads to an amelioration of symptoms. Surgical intervention, such as oophorectomy, should be avoided at all costs, since it may lead to problems from adhesions and exacerbate the situation.

Gynaecology 13

A 20-year-old single unemployed West Indian woman of Negro ancestry was seen as an emergency in the accident and emergency department at the request of her general practitioner. Her menarche had occurred at the age of 13 and she normally had regular periods with bleeding for 5 days every 29 days. She had been having regular intercourse without contraception, although she did not wish to become pregnant, and her last menstrual period had been 8 weeks before presentation. She had attended her GP 3 weeks previously complaining of increased vaginal discharge and was treated with Canesten (clotrimazole) pessaries and oral metronidazole. She complained at that time of nausea and breast tenderness, but was reassured that nothing was seriously wrong.

The morning of presentation she suddenly developed central chest pain, which was severe, and associated with several attacks of vomiting. She then became short of breath, and developed centralised abdominal pain. There was no cough, haemoptysis, palpitations, or vaginal bleeding. There had been no preceding dyspareunia.

The SHO in the A & E department thought she might have an ectopic pregnancy and referred her to the gynaecologist on duty. He found a distressed, dyspnoeic patient, who was pale and sweating. Her pulse was 120 beats/ minute, and blood pressure 85/52 mmHg. She was agitated and mildly confused. Cardiac auscultation revealed a gallop rhythm. The chest appeared normal, with good and equal air entry, and no adventitious sounds. The abdomen was diffusely tender. Vaginal examination showed that the uterus was mildly tender, but there were no adnexal masses, no cervical excitation, and no vaginal bleeding. The cervix was closed. Examination of the calves revealed no abnormality. She was afebrile.

1. Discuss the differential diagnosis.
2. Comment on the prescription of metronidazole three weeks before presentation.
3. What investigations would you perform?
4. Describe her further management.

1. Although the signs of shock which are manifest in this patient are consistent with the diagnosis of severe haemorrhage secondary to an ectopic pregnancy, the history does not suggest this condition. Intra-abdominal bleeding may cause irritation of the diaphragm, but this is associated with shoulder-tip referred pain, not central chest pain. Crushing central chest pain can occur secondarily to severe hypotension, but if this was due to haemorrhage from a damaged fallopian tube, it would almost certainly be preceded by abdominal pain. In addition, it is usually associated with air hunger, tachycardia (experienced as 'palpitations'), and clouding of consciousness. None of these occurred in the present case (air hunger is more dramatic than simple 'shortness of breath').

   The most likely cause of the symptoms and signs described above is a haemoglobinopathy, probably sickle cell disease (homozygous, HbSS). In this condition, the abnormal haemoglobin molecule reacts to hypoxia by taking on a 'sickle' shape, with loss of red cell flexibility. This leads to peripheral red cell sequestration, with small vessel occlusion and tissue infarction. The clinical seriousness of the condition is governed by the extent to which other haemoglobins, not normally prevalent in the adult, such as HbF_1 HbA_2 or HbC, can be produced by the individual and dilute the effects of the HbS. Stressful situations, such as early pregnancy, can precipitate attacks in previously unaffected individuals, although a history of previous attacks is usual. In the present case, close questioning revealed what sounded like a sickling crisis at the age of 14, precipitated by pneumonia. Presenting symptoms of a sickling crisis are shortness of breath, bone pain (often in the hands and legs) and chest pain. For obscure reasons, chest pain is the typical presentation in pregnancy.

   The other serious condition to be considered in pregnancy is thromboembolic disease. In the present case, there were no abnormal signs in the calves (swelling, heat, tenderness), or in the pelvis (tenderness, heat). There was no fever (a mild pyrexia is common with deep vein thrombosis) and no localising signs in the lungs. Acute pancreatitis is a very rare cause of chest pain, and should be excluded by appropriate investigation.

2. An increased colourless, non-irritant vaginal discharge is common in pregnancy and does not require treatment unless pathogens such as Trichomonas vaginalis can be demonstrated. The complaints of nausea and breast tenderness are merely signs indicating pregnancy.

3. The most urgent investigation is a haemoglobin estimation and sickle screen. Her haemoglobin was 9.4 g/dl and sickle test was positive (subsequent electrophoresis showed HbSC). The white count was $15.3 \times 10^9/l$. A pregnancy test was positive. Urea and electrolyte estimation showed urea 2.7 nmol/l; Na+ 37 nmol/l, K+ 3.3 nmol/l. An amylase of 230 u/l ruled out acute pancreatitis. Clotting factors were normal, with a platelet count of $350 \times 10^9/l$. Fibrin degradation products were not detected and the fibrinogen level was normal. Crisis can be precipitated by infection, but in this case HVS, MSU and blood cultures were all normal.

4. The priority in treatment is adequate oxygenation, usually given as 100% O_2 by face mask. Rehydration with intravenous colloids, such as normal saline or Hartmann's solution, is important to reduce blood viscosity. Treatments such as the use of intravenous bicarbonate or urea are not of proven benefit and are no longer used. Should the condition fail to improve with O_2 and rehydration, blood transfusion is used to 'dilute' the abnormal cells and improve the oxygen-carrying capacity of the blood in the peripheral tissues. If more than 2 units of blood are given, 'exchange transfusion' techniques should be used to prevent overload of the circulation. Any infection discovered should be treated vigorously with appropriate antibiotics.

Gynaecology 14

A 27-year-old housewife was using the combined oral contraceptive pill. She had a 'pill' withdrawal bleed on the 16th August but began to bleed again only 17 days into her next cycle of pills. She began to experience morning nausea and backache. Despite the fact that she had not missed taking any pills, she was anxious lest she had accidentally become pregnant, since a pregnancy would have posed financial problems for the couple at that particular time. Three 'home' pregnancy tests were, however, negative. Nonetheless, a gynaecologist whom she consulted privately diagnosed pregnancy and referred her to a pregnancy advisory service. At the clinic, the diagnosis of pregnancy was also confirmed on vaginal examination. She was admitted for a suction termination of pregnancy under general anaesthetic. Under anaesthetic the cervix was dilated to 10 mm and a Karman 8 suction cannula was inserted. However, no products of conception were found, and, instead, some fatty tissue was found blocking the cannula when it was withdrawn. Further examination revealed a normal sized uterus. Laparotomy confirmed a fundal perforation of the uterus.

1. Classify the reasons for accidental pregnancy while taking the combined oral contraceptive pill.
2. Explain the repeated diagnosis of pregnancy with the finding of an empty, normal sized uterus at operation.
3. What further investigations ought to have been done?
4. What are the dangers of perforation of the uterus with a suction cannula, and what action should be taken on discovery of the perforation?

1. The simplest reason for failure of the combined oral contraceptive to prevent pregnancy is for the woman to forget to take it. However, provided she takes the missed pill together with the next day's pill, the risk of failure for this single omission is quite small (unlike with the continuous low-dose, progestogen-only pill). The other reasons are interference with absorption and accelerated metabolism. Many factors may cause poor absorption, but the commonest is probably an episode of viral enteritis causing vomiting and/or diarrhoea. Broad-spectrum antibiotics, for example, given to treat a urinary tract infection, may disturb bowel flora and thus interfere with absorption. Accelerated metabolism is usually the result of administered drugs, notably antiepileptics such as barbiturates and phenytoin.

2. A not uncommon error in gynaecological diagnosis is to confuse an extrauterine pelvic tumour with enlargement of the uterus. Masses such as ovarian tumours, particularly if adherent to the uterus, can easily be misdiagnosed as a uterine fibroid. Another cause of error is a full bladder. It is, however, unlikely that the bladder would have been equally full on each occasion in this case, and an ovarian cyst is therefore the most likely cause of the mistaken diagnosis of uterine enlargement.

3. The simplest way of confirming the diagnosis would have been an ultrasound scan. This is a wise precaution in all cases where there is the slightest doubt about the diagnosis of pregnancy, or about the gestational age. The technique appropriate for termination of pregnancy varies with gestational age and so a precise knowledge of the age of the fetus is important to ensure safety.

4. The danger of uterine perforation with a suction cannula is that intra-abdominal contents such as the bowel may be damaged. This is more likely than with sounds or even a curette, since the bowel is actively sucked against the edge of the curette. When such a perforation is discovered, it is imperative that a laparotomy be performed to enable close inspection of the abdominal contents. This will include checking the bowel along its whole length for damage. Such close scrutiny is impossible using laparoscopy.

    In the case described, laparotomy revealed a 7.5 cm diameter cyst of the left ovary, lying in the pouch of Douglas. Ovarian cystectomy was attempted, but proved impossible, so a total oophorectomy was performed. Histology revealed a well differentiated endometrioid carcinoma of 'low malignant potential'. No addition treatment was given and repeat laparoscopies at 6, 18 and 30 months showed no evidence of recurrence.

Gynaecology 15

Mrs EM was a 34-year-old housewife and her husband a labourer. They had 3 children aged 14, 12 and 10. She had first attended the gynaecology clinic because of an abnormal cervical smear. At this time she did not have any gynaecological complaint and on examination the only abnormality was a small red area on the posterior lip of her cervix, which did not bleed on contact.

Colposcopic examination revealed cervical intraepithelial neoplasia grade III (CIN III; carcinoma in situ) which extended into the cervical canal. The upper limit of the lesion was not, however, visible.

A subsequent cervical cone biopsy revealed an area of infiltrative squamous carcinoma within the cervical canal. A diagnosis of a stage Ia (occult invasive) carcinoma of the cervix was therefore made and she was treated with three courses of intracavity caesium followed by a Wertheim's hysterectomy 6 weeks later. There was no evidence of invasive carcinoma in the hysterectomy specimen or lymph nodes. Some areas of severe dysplasia were, however, present and were noted to approach the excision line on the vaginal cuff. Smears from the vaginal vault were subsequently examined at 3-monthly intervals. These were normal until 18 months after the operation, when large numbers of malignant cells were observed in a routine smear.

There was no pelvic abnormality on routine examination, but colposcopy demonstrated a wide atypical transformation zone localised to the vaginal vault and a biopsy from this area showed features consistent with carcinoma in situ. There was no evidence of invasion.

1. What do you think is the most likely origin of this lesion?
2. How would you treat it?
3. What follow up would you advise?

1. Despite the radical therapy used for this patient's occult invasive cervical carcinoma, she was unfortunately found to have residual disease within 2 years of her initial treatment. The lesion observed at follow-up does not appear to have been recurrence of the original tumour. It probably arose from the residual dysplastic epithelium noted in the cut edge of the vaginal cuff obtained at hysterectomy (apparently missed during the colposcopy which preceded the operation).

   Although this is an unusual problem, the case nonetheless highlights the need for careful preoperative colposcopic assessment to determine the vaginal extent of the lesion and hence define the length of vagina that must be excised. (In the absence of colposcopic facilities, Schiller's iodine test is the only way in which upper vaginal involvement may be detected.) It also supports the concept that the aetiological factors which predispose to squamous cell carcinoma of the cervix may also act as carcinogenic stimuli on the vagina and emphasises the importance of prolonged follow-up (with special attention to the vagina) of all patients treated for cervical carcinoma.

2. In view of the localised nature of this patient's premalignant vaginal lesion and her age, further radical surgery, such as a partial or total vaginectomy, was not considered appropriate.

   Small areas of vaginal intraepithelial neoplasia of the type observed in this case are best treated using some form of local ablative therapy. Four methods are available, namely cryocautery, electrocautery, electrodiathermy and the carbon dioxide laser.

   Cryocautery and electrocautery are widely available and can be performed as outpatient procedures. These will only destroy tissue to a depth of 3 mm and this limits their use for cervical intraepithelial neoplasia, where gland crypt involvement to a greater depth may occur. This is not, however, a problem with lesions which are confined to the vaginal epithelium.

   Electrodiathermy destroys tissue more effectively, but usually requires general anaesthesia.

   Colposcopically guided laser therapy was used in this case. This technique can be used to destroy small areas of tissue (2 mm in diameter) with great precision to any required depth. It causes minimal discomfort and can also be performed as an outpatient procedure.

3. The patient was subsequently advised to have vaginal smears taken for cytological examination at 3-monthly intervals for 1 year, 6-monthly intervals for a further 2 years, and annually for life.

Gynaecology 16

A 17-year-old Negro woman, who lived in a small village in South Africa, presented as a gynaecological outpatient complaining of prolonged heavy periods associated with severe pain during menstruation. She had always experienced dysmenorrhoea during the first day of menstruation, which she described as 'gripping' in nature. This had, however, become more severe over the previous year, lasting for 2–3 days, and during the day before her period she experienced a suprapubic ache. She had never taken any medication for the pain. Her menarche had occurred 4 years earlier and her menstrual cycle had always been regular with bleeds of 4–6 days duration every 28–30 days. These had initially been scanty, but had gradually become heavier and longer. During the preceding 4–6 months she had passed large clots and her periods had lasted between 7 and 10 days. She denied having had sexual intercourse and had no other gynaecological symptoms.

On examination, her mucosae were pale but she was otherwise healthy in appearance. Abdominal examination revealed a mass arising from the pelvis consistent with a uterus of 14 weeks size. Vulval examination confirmed that she had an intact hymen and vaginal examination with one finger revealed that her cervix and vagina were normal. Her uterus was irregular and enlarged to approximately 12–14 weeks in size. It was firm in consistency and appeared to be enlarged by a right-sided fundal fibroid. There were no adnexal masses. Subsequent ultrasound examination confirmed these findings.

Haemoglobin measurement (9.2 g/dl) confirmed her clinical anaemia and a blood film showed this to be microcytic and hypochromic in nature. Her white cell count and ESR were normal.

A diagnostic curettage was performed on the 12th day of the cycle under general anaesthesia. Her uterine cavity was found to be 10 cm in length and appeared to be distorted by a right-sided fundal fibroid. The previous clinical findings were confirmed. Endometrial curettings, which were normal in appearance, were obtained. Because of her severe menorrhagia, anaemia and clinical findings, it was decided to perform a myomectomy.

At laparotomy the uterus was indeed irregularly enlarged with what appeared to be a 7–8 cm diameter fibroid on the right side. Both tubes and ovaries of the fundus were of normal appearance. After applying a Bonney's myomectomy clamp, an incision was made over the right anterior aspect of the uterus in an attempt to enucleate the fibroid. This proved to be difficult because no pseudocapsule could be identified and, with deep incision, the myometrium was found to be studded with brown-black cystic spaces of 1–2 mm diameter surrounded by thickened myometrium with a diffuse whorl-like trabecular pattern.

1. What is the diagnosis?
2. What is the aetiology of this condition?
3. How would you treat this patient?
4. What is her prognosis?

1. This young woman presents the typical clinical history and operative findings of uterine adenomyosis. In this case the abnormal tissue appeared to be localised to the right cornu of the uterus, forming a rounded swelling or adenomyoma. The aetiology of the condition is unknown, but histological examination reveals endometrial islands scattered through the myometrium, which shows hyperplastic and hypertrophic change. It is thought to arise as a result of downgrowths of the endometrium into the myometrium. These respond to the cyclical hormonal changes of the ovulatory cycle, which cause an accumulation of menstrual products within the gland 'lumen' giving rise to the blood-filled cystic spaces observed on incising the tissue.

2. Adenomyosis occurs most frequently in parous women over the age of 30 and is more common in its diffuse form, when it may be scattered throughout the myometrium. This type is often not suspected clinically, but is observed in up to 20% of hysterectomy specimens from women with a primary complaint of unexplained menorrhagia and who have only slight diffuse uterine enlargement.

   A solitary adenomyoma in a young woman within 4 years of the menarche is a rare event and, although fibroids are also rare at this age, it is understandable that this latter diagnosis should have been made in a woman with a localised uterine enlargement, menorrhagia, and who was found to have distortion of the uterine cavity. Dysmenorrhoea is common in women of this age and the history of increasingly severe dysmenorrhoea and premenstrual pain is more typical of adenomyosis than of an intramural fibroid. (It may, however, occur with expulsion of a submucous fibroid.)

3. A localised adenomyoma in a young woman can be excised, thus allowing reproductive function to be conserved. In older women, where no further children are desired, hysterectomy with conservation of the ovaries is undoubtedly the correct treatment.

   In the case described, an attempt was made to resect the abnormal tissue, but this was found to be very much more extensive than suspected from the uterine shape. A biopsy was therefore taken to confirm the diagnosis, the uterus was closed and long-term treatment with progestagens (norethisterone 5 mg daily) for 6 months was commenced. This resulted in moderate uterine involution (to approximately 8 weeks size) and a significant improvement in her dysmenorrhoea and menorrhagia. Danazol (antigonadotrophin) treatment, which was not available at the time, would perhaps have been preferable. Prostaglandin synthetase inhibitors (e.g. flufenamic acid) may have a therapeutic role in this condition, but because of the difficulty in achieving a certain diagnosis before hysterectomy, have not thus far been studied in a systematic fashion.

4. Hysterectomy is curative, but long-term prognosis is poor after conservative therapy. When appropriate, the patient should be encouraged to complete her family so that hysterectomy can be performed. Symptoms cease after the menopause and a conservative approach may be preferable during the perimenopausal period.

A housewife aged 34 years, who had experienced continuous painless vaginal bleeding for 2 months, was referred to the gynaecology clinic by her GP. During the first 2 weeks the blood loss had been extremely heavy, requiring her to use 10 or more tampons a day, and was bright red in colour with occasional clots. Her GP had therefore prescribed a 2-week course of norethisterone tablets 5 mg b.d., which had reduced the bleeding to a brown discharge requiring only one or two tampons each day. When she stopped these tablets the heavy bleeding recurred for 5 days and was followed by a persistent brown discharge, which appeared to be heavier when she used tampons than when she used sanitary towels.

Her menstrual cycle had previously been relatively regular with 4–5 days bleeding every 25–30 days. There was no history of postcoital bleeding and she and her husband were using sheaths for contraception. She had suffered from anorexia nervosa when 20 years old and since this time had occasionally taken tranquillisers. She was not taking any hormone preparation and was otherwise well.

There was no abnormality on general or abdominal examination. Pelvic examination revealed a normal-sized anteverted and mobile uterus and there were no adnexal masses. Her cervix and vulva were also healthy. Speculum examination of her vagina, however, revealed an ulcerated area in the mid portion of the posterior wall of her vagina. The ulcer, which was approximately 5 cm long and 1 cm wide, had clean but slightly rolled edges and appeared to be granulating centrally. She had no evidence of ulcers elsewhere on her body.

1. What is the diagnosis?
2. What investigations would you perform?

1. Vaginal ulceration may occur as a result of direct trauma from a foreign body (e.g. a ring pessary), venereal disease, chemical burns (e.g. potassium permanganate), or malignancy.

   Vaginal carcinoma usually occurs in women in their fifties. Bleeding is the commonest symptom associated with this condition, although an offensive purulent discharge may also be presented in advanced cases. These ulcers are usually friable and bleed with touch. Malignant growths in surrounding viscera, such as the rectum, bladder or urethra, may extend to the vagina and cause ulceration. Metastatic spread may also occur from the cervix, endometrium or ovary. Endometriosis of the rectovaginal septum can produce ulceration of the posterior vaginal wall, which is clinically indistinguishable from that due to malignancy, and syphilis and tuberculosis may both cause painless vaginal ulceration. The former usually has raised rolled edges while the latter causes an undermined discharging lesion.

   Herpes simplex, now the commonest cause of vulval ulceration, may occasionally cause vaginal ulceration, but rarely in isolation. Other rare venereal causes of vaginal ulceration include granuloma inguinale (due to *Corynebacterium granulomatis*), chancroid or soft sore (due to *Haemophilus ducreyi*) and lymphogranuloma venereum (due to *Chlamydia trachomatis*). These usually arise from the vulva and are painful. They are very rare in Europe and North America.

   Bechet's syndrome is a chronic relapsing condition characterised by recurrent ulceration of the mouth and genitalia. It is probably viral in origin and may cause isolated vulval, vaginal or cervical ulceration.

   Chronic douching with antiseptic solutions may cause vaginal ulceration and this should always be excluded by direct questioning.

   Tampon usage for more than three consecutive weeks has also been shown to be a cause of benign vaginal ulceration.

2. Biopsy must always be performed even when the ulcer has a benign appearance, as in this case. This will exclude primary and secondary malignancy and endometriosis. It may also be of help in the diagnosis of Bechet's syndrome (a vasculitis affecting small and medium-sized arteries and veins) and any of the inflammatory conditions listed, or may demonstrate granulation tissue containing 'foreign' fibres derived from tampons as in this case. A diagnostic curettage was performed to exclude an intrauterine cause for her abnormal bleeding.

   A differential white cell count and ESR may help to demonstrate an underlying inflammatory cause. Both were normal in this case.

   Syphilitic serology does not become positive until several weeks after the primary chancre has healed, but the spirochete (*Treponema pallidum*) can occasionally be identified by dark field examination of fluid from the chancre, or by immunofluorescent staining of a dried smear. Cultures for *Herpes simplex* and *Chlamydia trachomatis* should be sent in appropriate virus medium. *Haemophilus ducreyi* is difficult to culture and clinical diagnosis is more reliable than smears or cultures.

   Granuloma inguinale may be diagnosed by identifying Gram

negative bipolar rods with large mononuclear cells (Donovan bodies) in direct smears from the ulcer which have been treated with Giemsa or Wright's stains. Biopsy may also be helpful.

The site, linear nature, benign appearance and finding of tampon fibres in the granulation tissue obtained by biopsy in this case all supported a diagnosis of ulceration due to chronic tampon usage following an episode of dysfunctional uterine bleeding. The ulcer healed rapidly after the patient was advised not to use tampons. Serologic tests for syphilis at 6 weeks were negative.

Gynaecology 18

A 34-year-old unmarried doctor was referred for advice about her heavy periods. She had never been pregnant and had always had a regular 28-day menstrual cycle. Her periods lasted for only 5 days, but during the preceding year the bleeding had become so heavy that she was unable to go to work on the first day. She used approximately 40 sanitary towels for each period and frequently passed clots during the first 2 days. She experienced some cramping pain during her periods and had occasional discomfort low in her abdomen which was most marked on the left side. She had not experienced any intermenstrual bleeding and had never had intercourse. Fifteen months before, she had undergone a laparotomy at another hospital and a diagnosis of uterine fibromyomata (fibroids) had been made. A single pedunculated fundal fibroid had been removed, but as the remaining fibroids extended behind the bladder and into the left broad ligament, and as the patient wished to preserve her reproductive potential and had not agreed to hysterectomy, no attempt had been made to remove them.

She was an extremely slender woman and abdominal palpation revealed a firm 14 weeks size mass arising from the pelvis. Pelvic examination confirmed an irregular firm fibroid uterus of 14 weeks size with a cornual fibroid on the left side. There was no other pelvic abnormality. Her haemoglobin was 11.4 g/dl and a cervical smear was normal.

1. What treatment would you advise for this patient?
2. In what circumstances may uterine fibroids cause pain?
3. What advice would you give about contraception and pregnancy?
4. List the degenerative processes that may affect uterine fibroids.

1. Although a hysterectomy would eradicate this patient's menorrhagia and prevent recurrence of the fibroids, her age, marital status, nulliparity and desire to conserve her uterus make this inappropriate.

    Uterine fibromyomata are common tumours and although increased menstrual loss is common, the reason is often not clear unless the uterine cavity is enlarged by submucous fibroids. On the other hand, quite large tumours may develop without producing any change in menstruation. When severe menorrhagia occurs in association with relatively small fibroids, the possibility of concomitant dysfunctional uterine bleeding should always be borne in mind.

    Myomectomy is feasible in most cases but should not be attempted unless the patient is prepared to consent to a hysterectomy, as this may very occasionally be necessary to stop uncontrollable bleeding during the operation. The surgeon who performed her first laparotomy should have obtained consent for this procedure before embarking on a laparotomy.

    As this patient was very keen to avoid further surgery, she was treated initially with danazol 200 mg daily for 3 months. During treatment her menstruation effectively became normal, but the menorrhagia recurred immediately after this was stopped. As she found long-term drug therapy even less acceptable than surgery, a further laparotomy was performed. She understood and accepted the risk that hysterectomy might be required. Several intramural and subserous fibroids were removed and a round ligament plication performed to reduce the likelihood of small bowel adhesions to the incision on the anterior wall of the uterus. Her menstrual losses subsequently became acceptable.

    Other possible drug therapies include controlling the menstrual flow with progestagens such as medroxyprogesterone acetate (Provera), or the induction of an 'artificial menopause' with long-acting LHRH analogue (buserelin). This produces a substantial reduction in the size of fibroids (up to 50%), but the treatment carries all the disadvantages of the normal menopause (vasomotor instability, loss of calcium from the bones) and cannot therefore be maintained for longer than 6–12 months. Once the therapy is discontinued the fibroids rapidly regrow. However, buserelin therapy can be useful to reduce the size and vascularity of fibroids before myomectomy, thus making the procedure simpler and safer.

2. Pain is a relatively uncommon presenting feature in women with uterine fibromyomata. Congestive dysmenorrhoea may occur but is not usually severe. Pressure on surrounding viscera may produce pelvic discomfort, as in this case. Rarely, compression of nerves within the pelvis may cause pain radiating to the back and lower extremities. Subserous fibroids have relatively thick pedicles and rarely undergo torsion. However, when they do, their presentation mimics ovarian torsion and is that of 'an acute abdomen'. When submucous fibroids become pedunculated the uterus frequently attempts to expel the tumour. The resulting colicky pain, cervical dilatation and vaginal bleeding produce a clinical presentation which resembles a spontaneous abortion.

Acute haemorrhagic infarction (red degeneration) causes severe localised uterine pain, occurs most commonly during pregnancy, and may be confused with a concealed placental abruption. Infection and sarcomatous change may also cause pain, but are rare.

3. Fibroids are dependent on oestrogens for their growth and many gynaecologists therefore consider that oestrogen-containing oral contraceptives should not be used in these patients. Exogenous oestrogens, however, suppress endogenous oestrogen production and there is at present no evidence that combined oral contraceptives stimulate more rapid growth in uterine fibroids than would occur anyway. Provided that uterine size is checked regularly, the combined pill can therefore be used in women with fibroids and may, in fact, prove beneficial because of the reduced bleeding associated with pill withdrawal bleeds. Progestogen-only contraceptives may also be used.

   Intrauterine devices are contraindicated only when there is menorrhagia, or when distortion of the uterine cavity is suspected. Opinions differ on the advisability of vaginal delivery after myomectomy. In theory, if the endometrial cavity has been opened during the operation the scar carries a similar risk to that following classical caesarean section. In practice, however, myomectomy scars rarely rupture in labour, and a 'trial of scar' is not contraindicated on this basis alone.

4. The following types of benign degenerative processes may occur in uterine fibroids: atrophic (after pregnancy or menopause), hyaline, cystic, calcific, septic, carneous (red degeneration) and myxomatous. Malignant (sarcomatous) change occurs in less than 0.1% of diagnosed fibroids.

Gynaecology 19

A 38-year-old housewife attended a family planning clinic to have her intrauterine contraceptive device (IUCD) checked. Four years earlier, shortly after her second caesarean section, she had had a copper-bearing device inserted. This had been removed after a year because her husband had a vasectomy. Fourteen months later, having separated from her husband, she returned and requested a second intrauterine device. Another copper-bearing device was inserted without difficulty. Although she initially experienced intermenstrual bleeding for a month this subsequently stopped. Menstruation occurred every 28–30 days. It lasted for only 3 days and was not heavy. She missed her clinic appointments 6 and 12 months after the insertion, but returned at 14 months complaining of an intermittent thin watery offensive discharge of 3 months duration. She also complained of occasional discomfort in the right suprapubic region. This did not occur with menstruation and was not associated with any specific activity.

On examination she appeared healthy. There was no abnormality on abdominal examination. Vaginal examination revealed a malodorous, watery discharge which was greyish-white in colour. The cervix appeared to be healthy and the threads of the IUCD were visible. The uterus was of normal size, anteverted and mobile. There were no adnexal masses nor any pelvic tenderness. A cervical smear and high vaginal swab (HVS) were taken. These were reported as showing:

Cervical smear: no evidence of malignancy
HVS: Pus cells +
       Squames ++
       Gram negative rods ++++
       Gardnerella vaginalis isolated.

1. What is the significance of the HVS result?
2. What other investigation should this patient have had?
3. How would you manage this patient?

1. *Gardnerella vaginalis* vaginitis is now recognised as the third most common form of infective vaginitis in women in the reproductive age group. Previously termed *Haemophilus vaginalis* and then *Corynebacterium vaginale*, this Gram negative aerobic bacillus has recently been renamed after Gardner, who first recognised it as a vaginal pathogen. The discharge of which this patient complained is typical. The diagnosis is often missed, however, because the discharge is less florid than that associated with either *Candida albicans* or *Trichomonas vaginalis*, and overt vaginal inflammation and vulval irritation are both less common than with these latter infections. Wet preparations of the discharge characteristically contain so-called 'clue cells', which are epithelial cells covered with small Gram negative rods. Until recently, few laboratories have specifically attempted to culture the bacillus and in years past this patient would probably have been considered to have a 'non-specific' vaginitis.

2. Although an intrauterine device may produce a watery non-specific discharge, high vaginal swabs should be sent for culture and sensitivities in all women complaining of a vaginal discharge. In addition, a woman who requests reinsertion of an intrauterine contraceptive device a year after her husband has had a vasectomy should be considered to be at increased risk of sexually transmitted disease. Cervical swabs should, therefore, be taken and conveyed to the laboratory in Stewart's medium for anaerobic culture to exclude *Neisseria gonorrhoeae* infection.

3. A variety of treatments have been given to women with *Gardnerella vaginalis*. A mixture of three sulphonamides in a cream base (triple sulpha cream) can be applied locally and effects a cure in approximately 80% of cases. Oral tetracyclines and ampicillin have produced similar results. Recent experience, however, suggests that oral metronidazole in a dose of 400 mg three times daily for a week is the best therapy, effecting a cure in approximately 95% of patients. Although metronidazole displays activity against *Gardnerella vaginalis* in vitro it has been suggested that its efficacy in vivo reflects an interaction between vaginal anaerobic bacteria (e.g. *Bacteroides fragilis* and *Bacillus melaninogenicus*) and *Gardnerella vaginalis*. This is because these vaginal anaerobes appear to inhibit phagocytosis of aerobic bacteria by leukocytes and may facilitate pathogenic growth of *Gardnerella*.
    Occasional episodes of unilateral suprapubic discomfort are not uncommon in IUCD users. The cause of this discomfort is uncertain, but probably reflects uterine contractions precipitated by the device. At the time of menstruation this pain may also be due to retrograde flow of small amounts of menstrual blood into the peritoneal cavity. Although salpingitis is 3–6 times more common in IUCD users (especially those who are promiscuous) and may be unilateral, it is usually associated with a persistent severe suprapubic pain, malaise, and abdominal and pelvic tenderness. In more severe cases there is usually a marked pyrexia, rebound tenderness, cervical excitation pain and a tubal swelling (due to a pyosalpinx) may also be palpable. This patient had no evidence of salpingitis.

Gynaecology 20

A 19-year-old single civil service clerk attended the gynaecology outpatient clinic complaining of a white vaginal discharge of 18 months duration. This was associated with vulval irritation, but had a normal odour. Her menarche had occurred at the age of 13 years, but her periods had been irregular with a 4–6 weeks cycle until she had started on the oral contraceptive pill at the age of 18 years.

She had become aware of her discharge 6 months before starting the pill. It also preceded her first sexual contact. Two months after having intercourse she developed, in addition, a vulval pruritis. Her doctor, who did not examine her at this time, diagnosed a 'thrush' infection and prescribed clotrimazole vaginal pessaries. After she had completed this treatment the vulval irritation stopped, but the white discharge persisted and she occasionally had to wear a 'panty liner' to prevent staining of her underwear. Her doctor had subsequently prescribed oral metronidazole and ketoconazole, but without any beneficial effect. Her pill withdrawal bleeds occurred every 28 days and there was no history of postcoital or breakthrough bleeding. She had a regular boyfriend. She had never been pregnant and had no relevant past medical history.

On examination she was a fit young woman. There was no abnormality of her breasts nor abdomen. Her vulva looked normal. Speculum examination revealed a normal cervix. There was a moderate amount of white vaginal discharge, but no inflammation. Her uterus was of normal size, axial and mobile. No adnexal masses were palpable and there was no pelvic tenderness.

1. What investigations would you perform?
2. What is the most likely cause of her discharge?
3. What advice would you give her?

1. To prescribe treatment for a vaginal discharge without examining the patient is inexcusable. *Candida albicans* is a yeast which characteristically causes a thick, curd-like white discharge, which is frequently adherent to the vaginal skin. It may produce a red raw vulva and vagina, or alternatively it may be associated with a whitish discharge of normal appearance. There is frequently pruritis and some soreness. *Trichomonas vaginalis* usually produces a severe vaginitis with, classically, a malodorous yellow-green frothy discharge. This may occasionally be blood-stained. It causes vulvovaginal erythema and oedema and marked vulval soreness. In the most severe form there are petechial haemorrhages and swollen vaginal papillae, which give rise to the so-called 'strawberry vagina'. In mild cases there may, however, only be a slight increase in vaginal discharge. Microscopic examination of a wet preparation may reveal the causative motile protozoa. Although it is often possible to diagnose both of these infections in their florid forms by clinical examination alone, atypical presentation is not uncommon and mixed infections may occur. High vaginal swabs should therefore be sent for culture and microscopy, to confirm the diagnosis. It is also important to exclude *Gardnerella vaginalis*, the cause of so-called 'non-specific' vaginitis, and anaerobic bacteria such as *Bacteroides* sp. A cervical smear should also be sent to exclude malignancy. In addition both *Candida* and *Trichomonas* may be visible with Papanicolau staining.

2. The history and findings in this patient are strongly suggestive of a physiological discharge or 'leukorrhoea'. This is more common in women using combined oral contraceptives, possibly because of increased cervical secretions and vaginal desquamation. Leukorrhoea is typically non-adherent, abundant and white. Pruritis and slight discomfort may occur, either because of chafing, or the attempts of the patient to rid herself of the discharge using soap, deodorants or douching. Sexual excitement may cause an increased physiological discharge and it may also occur in the unduly tense or anxious woman. Concern that a discharge has a pathological cause may arise from adverse comments made by the patient's partner after sexual intercourse or cunnilingus. This may lead to overzealous use of soap, deodorants or douching, all of which may then precipitate a chemical vaginitis. Tight clothing or nylon underwear may also cause chafing and vulval soreness in a woman with a normal discharge. Rarely, a non-specific maladorous discharge may result from a foreign body in the vagina, such as a forgotten tampon or diaphragm.

3. The patient should always be questioned carefully to determine whether any of the above predisposing factors are present and advised accordingly. It must also be remembered that the mild pruritis resulting from a slightly increased physiological discharge may lead to scratching and excoriation which in turn precipitates itching and further scratching, frequently while asleep. Measures to break this chronic 'scratch-itch' cycle include wearing cotton pants in bed at night and even cotton gloves. Mild corticosteroid creams may also be beneficial, but should only be used for a few days as prolonged use may lead to atrophic changes in the vulval skin.

The HVS and cervical smear obtained from this patient were normal and simple reassurance was all that was required to solve her problem. It is seldom necessary to stop the oral contraceptive pill in women with this complaint.

Gynaecology 21

A 37-year-old housewife who was married to a teacher went to her GP for a cervical smear. The report stated that there were 'some fragments of abnormal epithelium, derived from squamous metaplasia, showing dyskaryosis and loss of differentiation. Advise referral for colposcopy'. She was therefore seen in the gynaecology clinic, where it was noted that she had two children, aged 15 and 17 years, by a previous marriage. Her periods occurred every 21 days and lasted for 3–4 days. She had no gynaecological complaints. She and her husband were using sheaths for contraception. She had never had any operation or serious illness.

She appeared fit and there was no abnormality on general examination. Her breasts and abdomen were also normal. Her vulva and vagina were normal. Speculum examination revealed a macroscopically normal cervix. Her uterus was of normal size, anteverted and mobile. There were no pelvic masses.

Her cervix was examined using a colposcope (x 10 magnification). The entire squamocolumnar junction (transformation zone) was visible with a small area of punctation on the posterior lip. Staining with acetic acid revealed white epithelium covering a similar area of the posterior lip of the cervix. Normal columnar epithelium was visible within the endocervical canal.

1. What is the significance of these changes?
2. How would you manage this patient?
3. What is the aetiology and prognosis of this lesion?

1. Dyskaryotic cells arise from dysplastic squamous epithelium at the squamocolumnar junction (transformation zone). This epithelium is characteristically hyperplastic and individual cells display a variable increase in the nuclear: cytoplasmic ratio (nuclear pleomorphism), number of mitotic figures and density of nuclear chromatin. When such cells are visualised in a cervical smear they indicate that the epithelium somewhere on the cervix is abnormal. Whether this change involves the full thickness of the epithelium (severe dysplasia/carcinoma-in-situ), or partial thickness (mild/moderate dysplasia) can only be determined by histological examination of the epithelium from which the abnormal cells have been obtained with the Ayre's spatula. The numbers of dyskaryotic cells and the severity of the nuclear pleomorphism do, however, give a clue as to the severity of the lesion.

   In an attempt to clarify the confused classification of epithelial changes in this condition, the term 'cervical intraepithelial neoplasia' (CIN) has been introduced. CIN III (or 3) indicates that the full thickness of the epithelium shows failure of differentiation with marked nuclear pleomorphism and multiple mitotic figures. This term embraces, and is synonymous with, three older histological terms: severe dysplasia, carcinoma-in-situ (CIS) and intraepithelial carcinoma.(IEC). CIN II (or 2) is synonymous with moderate dysplasia and CIN I (or 1) with mild dysplasia. (This latter change may also be observed in cervicitis.) The cytologist may use these histological terms to indicate the histological appearance of the epithelium from which (s)he thinks these cells originate; but cannot be certain of the diagnosis until full thickness cervical epithelium is obtained from the affected area and subjected to histological examination. Colposcopy makes it much easier to identify the affected area and therefore to obtain appropriate biopsies. Its usefulness depends on the fact that abnormal epithelium is supplied by abnormal blood vessels. The vessels are wider than normal, form loops between the epithelial rete pegs, and run closer to the surface than usual. On colposcopic examination, these vessels present a stippled appearance termed 'punctation'. In more advanced lesions the vessels run parallel to the surface and give rise to a 'mosaic' appearance. Branching vessels running close to the epithelial surface are suggestive of invasive carcinoma.

   Staining with acetic acid causes the dysplastic epithelium to assume an opaque appearance, so-called 'white epithelium'. This is a reversible change which reflects the increased cellular chromatin content.

2. Provided the whole of the transformation (also called transition) zone is visible, colposcopy makes it possible to identify and take punch biopsies from areas of abnormal cervical epithelium. If histological examination of this tissue shows that the basement membrane is intact (i.e. microinvasion can be excluded), then the abnormal epithelium can be destroyed using colposcopically guided local destructive techniques. The simplest, and most widely used, of these is cryocautery. So-called 'cold cautery', in which the epithelium is heated to 100°C, is, however, gaining popularity as there is less trouble with vaginal discharge after

treatment compared with cryocautery. These methods, although less radical than diathermy cautery, have the major advantage that they can be used on an outpatient basis. Laser vaporisation, although expensive, is also widely used. It enables abnormal epithelium to be destroyed with pin-point accuracy to a precise depth. It can be used on an outpatient basis and does not usually require analgesia.

The biopsies obtained from this patient confirmed CIN III, which was treated with cryocautery.

If the upper limit of the lesion cannot be seen, then a cervical cone biopsy must be obtained. Normal cervical epithelium contains glycogen and stains a mahogany colour with aqueous iodine solution (Schiller's test). Abnormal (and columnar) epithelium does not stain. The colposcopist can therefore use the appearance of the iodine-stained cervix to describe to the surgeon the width of the cone that he must obtain.

3. The most important aetiological factors in squamous carcinoma of the cervix are early age of coitus and number of sexual partners. Several infective agents have been implicated. Herpes virus type II and *Chlamydia trachomatis* are now thought to be unimportant in this regard. Human papilloma virus (types 16 and 18) are probably more significant.

Complete cure of early lesions, such as that seen in this patient, is usually achieved by simple local destructive therapy. Repeat cervical smears should be examined 3 and 6 months after treatment and annually thereafter in any woman who has had CIN, so that any recurrences will be detected early and can be retreated.

Gynaecology 22

A 52-year-old housewife was admitted as an emergency complaining of heavy vaginal bleeding for 7 weeks. Her general practitioner, who had not examined her, had prescribed oral progestogens the previous day, but as the bleeding had persisted he had referred her for an urgent assessment. Closer questioning revealed that she had experienced very irregular vaginal bleeding for several months. As this bleeding had followed 3 months of amenorrhoea she had chosen to assume that it was due to 'the change' and had not sought advice until it had become persistent. She also admitted to frequent postcoital bleeding and an offensive vaginal discharge for 4 months. She had not experienced any pain during the bleeding, or with intercourse. Her menstrual cycle had previously been regular with 7 days bleeding every 28–30 days. Her doctor had prescribed a combined oral contraceptive pill for her between the ages of 41 and 46 years. She had not used any contraception since stopping the pill and was not taking any drugs or hormonal preparations. She had not experienced any flushes. Her 6 children were aged between 12 and 32 years and had all been born normally. There was no other gynaecological complaint nor any significant past medical history. She had never had an operation. She smoked 20 cigarettes each day.

On examination she appeared anaemic and blood was therefore taken and sent for a haemoglobin estimation. There was no other abnormality on general examination, nor on examination of her breasts or abdomen. Vulval and vaginal examination revealed some old blood. The cervix was virtually replaced by a 2–3 cm diameter friable papilliferous tumour, which bled profusely when touched. Her uterus was retroverted, apparently normal in size, regular in outline and freely mobile. There were no adnexal masses. The tumour which was biopsied appeared on combined rectal and vaginal examination to extend for approximately 1 cm into the posterior vaginal vault, but not into the deep parametrial tissues.

Her haemoglobin result was 7.8 g/dl. The cervical biopsy was reported to consist of 'superficial fragments of non-keratinising squamous cell carcinoma with some areas of necrosis'.

1. What further investigations would you perform?
2. Describe the mode of spread of this tumour.
3. Describe the clinical staging of cervical carcinoma. Assuming that the above findings are confirmed, what stage would you assign in this patient?
4. What treatment would you advise?
5. What is her prognosis?

1. When a lesion is visible on the ectocervix, a punch (or wedge) biopsy must be taken to confirm or exclude a carcinoma. Colposcopy and cone biopsy are reserved for patients with abnormal cytology and no gross lesion. There is a high incidence of negative cervical smears in women with invasive carcinoma, as much of the tumour may be necrotic and obscure the abnormal cells. Cytology cannot be relied on to confirm or exclude the diagnosis of invasive carcinoma of the cervix.

   When the histological diagnosis has been confirmed, a full haematological and biochemical profile should be obtained. This must include a blood urea estimation and liver function tests. A chest X-ray and intravenous urogram (IVU) should also be performed. The patient should then be prepared for examination under anaesthesia (EUA) and cystoscopy, which are necessary to stage the tumour correctly. Sigmoidoscopy may also be necessary. Pelvic lymphangiography is advocated by some gynaecologists, but most consider it to be unreliable.

2. The tumour may be ulcerative, infiltrating, or exophytic as in this case. It may extend directly down the vagina, into the parametrium, myometrium, or into the bladder or rectum. Lymphatic spread involves the pelvic lymphatic chain (paracervical, obturator, and hypogastric nodes). Subsequent spread to the common iliac, para-aortic or inguinal nodes may occur in advanced disease. Haematogenous spread is infrequent.

3. Cervical cancer is staged according to the FIGO (International Federation of Gynaecology and Obstetrics) classification. Stage 0 is intraepithelial. Stage 1 is invasive carcinoma confined to the cervix. It includes microinvasion [stage Ia(i)], where the tumour penetrates less than 3 mm beyond the basement membrane, occult invasive [stage Ia(ii)], where the depth of invasion exceeds 3 mm, and stage Ib in which the tumour is clinically overt. In stage IIa the cancer involves the upper vagina and in stage IIb there is parametrial involvement. In stage IIIa the tumour reaches the lower vagina and in stage IIIb there is either extension to the pelvic side wall, hydronephrosis or a non-functioning kidney. Stage IVa indicates spread to adjacent organs (bladder or rectum) and stage IVb distant spread.

   Pelvic nodes are involved in 15% of stage I tumours, 25% of stage II, 50% of stage III and 66% of stage IV.

   This patient had a normal IVU, and EUA and cystoscopy confirmed the diagnosis that had been made on admission, of a stage IIa squamous carcinoma.

4. Most patients are treated with radiotherapy using caesium sources that are placed within the cervical canal and endometrial cavity, and at the vaginal vault (so called intracavitary irradiation). Under general anaesthesia, delivery systems which fit the uterine cavity and vagina are inserted. These are held in place with packing and their position is confirmed on X-ray. This enables isodose curves to be calculated for various areas of the pelvis. The actual radiation sources are only inserted if the position of the delivery system is satisfactory. This technique, which is known as 'afterloading', minimises unnecessary irradiation of the patient's attendants. Two

or three treatments at intervals of about 2–4 weeks are usual. These are combined with external irradiation, which is generally administered using megavoltage equipment in fractionated doses over 6–7 weeks. The bladder and rectum are protected using the central shield and a dose of approximately 5000 rad is directed at the pelvic lymph nodes.

In some young patients with stage Ib or IIa disease, a radical or Wertheim's hysterectomy with pelvic lymphadenectomy is preferred. This involves dissection of the ureters and removal of the upper third of the vagina and all lateral parametrial tissue. The ovaries and a functional vagina can, however, be conserved. Ureteric fistula, resulting from devascularisation of the ureter, is the major complication of radical surgery and occurs in approximately 3% of cases. Shortening of the vagina is seldom troublesome.

Many oncologists favour a combination of preoperative intracavitary irradiation followed by Wertheim's hysterectomy and pelvic lymphadenectomy. If the lymph nodes that are removed contain residual tumour, external beam therapy can then be directed at the pelvic side wall. This is the treatment that was used in this patient.

5. The prognosis of cervical carcinoma is closely related to the clinical staging of the disease. The following are approximate figures for 5-year survival: stage I 90%; stage II 60–80%; stage III 35–40% and stage IV 15%. The overall survival is about 50–60%.

Gynaecology 23

A 46-year-old publisher's secretary was referred for a gynaecological opinion because of a single episode of intermenstrual bleeding. She had never married nor been pregnant. Although she had had a regular sexual partner for some years, she had never used contraception and had not experienced any postcoital bleeding. Her menstrual cycle was regular with 3–4 days bleeding at intervals of 26–28 days. She had never experienced flushes and did not have any other relevant symptoms. Her last cervical smear, 9 years earlier, had been normal. A benign mass had been removed from her left breast in the same year. She had no other significant past medical history and was not taking any medication.

General examination was normal. There was a scar over her left breast, but no other abnormality. Abdominal palpation was normal. Her vulva and vagina were also of normal appearance. A cervical 'polyp' of approximately 5 mm diameter was, however, noted to be protruding from the external cervical os. A cervical smear was taken and the polyp was avulsed with polypectomy forceps. Bimanual palpation revealed a uterus which was of normal size, anteverted and mobile. There were no adnexal masses. She was discharged from the clinic, but told to return should she experience any further bleeding. The cervical smear was reported as 'negative'. Fourteen months later she attended her general practitioner for another cervical smear. She had no complaints and on passing a speculum he was rather surprised to see a fleshy red mass, approximately 2 cm long and 1 cm in diameter arising from her cervix. There was no contact bleeding when he took the smear and bimanual examination confirmed that the mass was soft and fleshy in consistency.

1. What is the most likely diagnosis?
2. Comment on her previous management.
3. What advice would you give this anxious patient?
4. What other symptoms may occur?

1. This neoplasm is almost certainly a benign endocervical polyp. These common tumours usually arise as a result of focal hyperplasia of the endocervix. They are usually covered by columnar epithelium and their stroma is composed of fibrous connective tissue containing numerous small blood vessels. Metaplastic change is frequent and inflammation with necrosis of the tip or even the whole polyp is typical. Their cause is unknown, but as they may occur in association with endometrial hyperplasia and endometrial polyps, it has been suggested that they may represent an abnormal local response to oestrogens. Other possible causes include localised congestion of cervical blood vessels and chronic cervicitis.

2. Metaplastic change in cervical polyps is common, but malignant change is rare. Despite this any polyp that is avulsed should be sent for histological examination and this was not done in this case. Polyps may coexist with an endometrial carcinoma and it cannot be assumed that they are the cause of any abnormal vaginal bleeding; a diagnostic dilatation and curettage should always be performed.

3. The recurrence of an endocervical polyp in this patient probably resulted from failure to perform endometrial and endocervical curettage in the first instance. She should, therefore, be advised to have a dilatation and curettage.

4. Intermenstrual and postcoital bleeding are the commonest symptoms. Post menopausal bleeding may also occur. Leukorrhoea, or an offensive infected discharge are also common.

Gynaecology 24

A suicidally depressed, very vague and weepy 83-year-old widow was admitted to a medical ward complaining of 'burning' dysuria and frequency for two weeks. Culture of a midstream urine specimen yielded a heavy growth of *Escherichia coli* and treatment with oral ampicillin 250 mg q.i.d. was started. After four days of treatment she was still complaining bitterly of dysuria and frequency and for the first time mentioned that she had noticed intermittent bleeding from her 'front passage' during the previous three weeks. There had been no other vaginal bleeding since her menopause. When the medical registrar performed a vaginal examination he was somewhat surprised to find a purple swelling of approximately 2 cm diameter replacing the external urethral meatus. He therefore sought the opinion of a gynaecologist. The only drugs that the patient had received were antidepressants and antibiotics that had been prescribed when she was admitted. There was no abnormality on general or abdominal examination. Vulval inspection confirmed the periurethral mass. The vulva, vagina, cervix and uterus were all atrophic and there were no pelvic masses.

1. What is the most likely diagnosis and the differential diagnosis?
2. How would you manage this patient?

1. A slight 'sliding' prolapse of the mucosa of the posterior urethral meatus often occurs to a minor degree in postmenopausal women. This is part of the process of urogenital atrophy which results from oestrogen deficiency. Physical 'trauma' (due to friction) may cause an exquisitely tender granulomatous swelling to develop in this prolapsed mucosa. This lesion, which is called a 'urethral caruncle', is much smaller than that seen in this patient (caruncles are usually less than 5 mm in diameter). She had a 'true' chronic urethral prolapse involving a complete annular aversion of the lower urethral mucosa. This also occurs as a result of oestrogen deficiency in elderly women. The cystitis suffered by this patient may have caused her to strain excessively while passing urine, thus accentuating a pre-existing minor degree of urethral prolapse. This probably led to strangulation of the prolapse, causing it to become grossly oedematous and haemorrhagic. The resulting tumour can easily be confused with a vulval, vaginal or lower urethral carcinoma.

2. This prolapse was treated by excising the thrombosed, haemorrhagic tissue and reconstituting the external urethral meatus. Care was taken to ensure that adequate mucosa was retained to reform the urethral opening without undue tension. As these patients frequently experience difficulty with micturition after surgery, an indwelling Foley catheter (made of silastic) was inserted and left in situ for 7 days. Urinary antiseptics were administered during this time and for 48 hours after removing the catheter.

Gynaecology 25

A 28-year-old housewife with two children aged 6 and 2 years was referred to the gynaecology clinic because of a vulval swelling. She had first noticed this 5 years earlier, after the birth of her first child. It had never caused her any problem and she therefore ignored it. No comment had been made about the swelling during her second pregnancy. Two months before referral the swelling had become painful and inflamed and had enlarged considerably. Her general practitioner had prescribed ampicillin and following this the inflammation had resolved. The swelling had, however, remained larger than before and was described as the size of a large grape. Both her pregnancies had been uncomplicated and her children had been born normally. The only significant past medical history was a cholecystectomy 2 years earlier.

There was no abnormality on general or abdominal examination. On parting the labia a 2 cm diameter swelling was apparent immediately posterior to the external urethral meatus extending upwards under the anterior vaginal wall. This was fluctuant and non-tender.

Her vulval, vagina and cervix were otherwise normal. Bimanual examination revealed a normal size, anteverted, mobile uterus and no pelvic mass.

1. What is the most likely cause of this swelling and what treatment would you advise?
2. What other cystic swellings may arise in the vulva and how would you treat them?

1. This patient had a paraurethral cyst. These arise as a result of blockage of the duct of a paraurethral (Skene's) gland. Such cysts frequently become infected, as in this case. They are usually less than 2 cm in diameter, but may enlarge up to 4 cm. If small and asymptomatic they are best ignored. Excision is justified when the cyst is large, or there is a history of infection. The cyst can be very difficult to remove as they frequently extend up under the anterior vaginal wall and prove to be much larger than expected. Great care has to be taken to avoid damage to the attenuated urethral mucosa which overlies the cyst.

2. The commonest vulval cyst is that which arises from blockage of the duct of Bartholin's (greater vestibular) gland. These glands lie deep to the posterior third of the labium majus (just inferior and lateral to the bulbocavernosus muscle). Their ducts open into the lateral aspect of the vulva adjacent to the vagina and just below the hymen. Gonorrhoea is an important cause of duct obstruction, but inspissated mucus and congenital narrowing also predispose to blockage. Reforming the duct opening by so called marsupialisation is the treatment of choice for both infected and non-infected cysts as it is simple and preserves the function of the gland. If the duct blocks and the cyst reforms after marsupialisation, then excision of the gland should be undertaken as an interval procedure. This is usually a very difficult operation because of the extremely rich blood supply with which the vulva is endowed. For this reason it is best avoided as a primary procedure for the non-infected cyst and should never be attempted if the cyst is infected.

   Cysts of epidermal origin (dermal inclusion cysts) may arise when skin is buried inadvertently during suture of an episiotomy, or during a vaginal repair operation. These should be excised if troublesome.

   Vulval skin contains a plentiful supply of sebaceous glands and apocrine sweat glands. The occlusion of a duct leading from a sebaceous gland results in an accumulation of sebaceous material forming a sebaceous cyst. Non-infected cysts may be excised; acutely infected cysts should be incised and drained. The apocrine sweat glands become functional after puberty. A benign cystic tumour may arise in a single gland forming a so-called hidradenoma. Rarely, occlusion of the ducts of multiple glands may occur producing an extremely pruritic microcystic condition called Fox-Fordyce disease.

   Cysts arising from Mullerian duct vestiges (Gartners' duct cysts) rarely extend to the vulva.

   Supernumerary mammary tissue arising in the vulval 'milk line' has been reported to form cysts during pregnancy, but this is excessively rare.

Gynaecology 26

A 68-year-old widow presented in the gynaecology clinic complaining that there was 'a lump in her front passage'. This had first appeared some 3–4 years earlier while she was nursing her husband, who had subsequently died of lung cancer. She was particularly aware of the lump 'coming down' when she was walking and straining and was constantly sore because it chafed against her underwear. There was no difficulty with micturition or defaecation and she had not experienced any vaginal discharge or bleeding. Her only pregnancy had been a miscarriage at the age of 37 years, 3 years after her marriage. She was a non-smoker and did not have a cough. A hysterectomy had been performed 22 years earlier because of menorrhagia due to fibroids and she had also undergone surgery for a peptic ulcer at the age of 50 years. She was taking analgesics for osteoarthritis of her spine, but was not on any other medication.

On examination she looked healthy and was not overweight. Her breasts and abdomen were normal apart from two operation scars. There were moderate atrophic changes of the vulva and protruding through the hymenal ring was a partial inversion of the vagina. There appeared to be only a minor degree of cystocoele and rectocoele. The swelling, which was the size of a small tangerine, appeared to arise from the vaginal vault and to contain bowel. There was no pelvic mass nor any evidence of stress incontinence.

1. What is this swelling?
2. What examination should have been performed to confirm this?
3. What treatment would you advise?

1. This patient has an enterocoele or vaginal vault prolapse following total hysterectomy — probably a form of incisional hernia. It may, at first sight, be confused with a rectocoele. The two conditions can usually be distinguished by combined rectal and vaginal examination, especially with the patient standing.

2. An enterocoele produces a reducible thickening or bulge of the upper rectovaginal septum. If the anterior vaginal wall is retracted with a Sims' speculum, the finger in the vagina can be used to delineate the extent of a rectocoele. If there is any doubt, a proctoscopic light source can be passed into the rectum; this will transilluminate a rectocoele, but not an enterocoele. Very occasionally peristalsis of bowel may be seen through a thin-walled enterocoele sac. Lateral pelvic X-rays obtained during barium studies of the small bowel for other purposes may occasionally reveal prolapse of ileum into the enterocoele.

3. If a ring pessary is retained, it may be suitable as a short-term measure in some patients. In the longer term, all patients, except for the very frail, should be treated surgically. This can be done by either the vaginal or the abdominal route. The vaginal approach, which is only suitable if there is a lax vagina, involves dissection and excision of the enterocoele sac, followed by apposition of the uterosacral ligaments. Redundant anterior and posterior vaginal wall skin is then excised and an anterior colporrhaphy and colpoperineorrhaphy performed. If the vagina is already narrowed, then colposuspension by the abdominal approach is preferable. A laparotomy is performed and the apex of the vagina identified. A subperitoneal 'tunnel' is then made around the lateral pelvic wall on each side, meeting up with an incision over the middle third of the sacrum to the left of the sigmoid mesocolon. Mersilene tape is attached to the vaginal vault, passed through the subperitoneal 'tunnels' and fixed to the presacral fascia. The major complication of this approach is persistent bleeding from the veins of the presacral plexus, which can be difficult to stop as the veins retract into their bony canals in the sacrum and are impossible to suture. Local pressure, or even the use of a pack removed as a secondary procedure, is usually the only way to stop the bleeding. Care should therefore be taken to make sure that blood is crossmatched and available before starting the procedure.

   It is important to remember that, in the erect posture, the vagina is virtually horizontal. Operative correction, by either approach, should always aim to restore the normal vaginal axis. Techniques that suspend the vaginal vault from the anterior abdominal wall should be avoided because they bring the vagina too far forward. This creates a hiatus posteriorly and promotes the recurrence of the enterocoele.

   Recurrent prolapse following vaginal repair can be treated either by the abdominal approach, or by sacrospinous fixation. This involves opening the vault of the vagina, dissecting around the right side of the sigmoid colon and suspending the vault of the vagina with a non-absorbable suture to a point on the sacrospinous ligament one-third of the way from the ischial spine to the sacrum. The major complication of this approach is perforation of the sigmoid colon.

Occasionally, obliteration of the vagina (Le Fort's operation) under local or regional anaesthesia, is indicated in a very old, frail patient.

In the case described above an abdominal colposuspension was performed, with a good result.

A nurse, married to an electrician, requested sterilisation. She was 32 years old and her husband was aged 35 years. They had two children, aged 7 and 5 years; both delivered by caesarean section because of cephalopelvic disproportion. She had used oral contraception before and after the delivery of her first child, but after the second baby had opted for an intrauterine contraceptive device. A Lippes loop size 'D' had been inserted in the postnatal clinic and she had initially been happy with this method of contraception, despite the fact that her periods became a lot heavier. During the year preceding presentation, however, her menstrual losses had become both prolonged and much heavier, with 9 days bleeding every 26–31 days. She passed large clots on the second and third day of bleeding and had decided that she could no longer cope with the IUCD. She had also experienced pain in the left lower abdomen and a sensation of 'something' in her pelvis. The pain occurred intermittently throughout the menstrual cycle, but was worse during periods and coitus. She had not experienced any intermenstrual or postcoital bleeding and had a normal vaginal discharge. Her general health was good and there was no relevant past medical or family history.

She looked healthy and there was no abnormality on general examination. Her breasts and abdomen were also normal. Pelvic examination, however, revealed a firm left adnexal mass of about 12 cm diameter which could not, with certainty, be separated from the uterus. The right ovary was not palpable.

It was therefore decided to perform a laparotomy and consent was obtained for hysterectomy should this prove necessary. At operation the uterus was found to be of normal size, axial and mobile. The left ovary was of normal appearance, but was adherent to a large friable mass which was contained within the left broad ligament and extended to involve the left fallopian tube. There was a tubo-ovarian mass of approximately 5–6 cm diameter on the right side; this appeared to be of infective origin. In order to ensure complete removal of this apparently malignant tumour a total abdominal hysterectomy and bilateral salpingo-oophorectomy were performed. Histological examination of the broad ligament mass showed it to be an 'endodermal sinus tumour' entirely separate from the ovary, which was normal.

1. What is this tumour and what marker does it produce?
2. How do you think this tumour may have arisen?
3. What other gynaecological tumours produce a marker?

1. The endodermal sinus tumour is a germ cell tumour of yolk sac origin. It usually secretes alpha-fetoprotein (AFP), which can be demonstrated either in the tumour using immunoperoxidase staining, or directly by measurement of plasma levels. This relatively rare malignant tumour, which usually occurs in young women, has a very poor prognosis with a reported median survival time of only 8 months. Fortunately, it is very chemosensitive and in women with residual tumour, or evidence of intraperitoneal spread, combination therapy with vincristine, cyclophosphamide and actinomycin has greatly improved the outlook.

2. The germ cells which differentiate approximately 3 weeks after conception (5 weeks gestation) develop in the root of the yolk sac ventrally and about 5 weeks later migrate by amoebic movement via the hindgut mesentery (probably by chemotaxis) to the genital ridges dorsally and come to lie within the cortex of the primitive ovary which is derived from the coelomic epithelium. The totally extragonadal site of the tumour in this patient suggests that some of the germ cells involved in this early embryonic migration remained separate from the gonad and came to lie within the broad ligament in which they subsequently underwent malignant change. AFP is also secreted by some teratomas (dermoid cysts).

3. Choriocarcinoma, a rare malignant tumour which occurs in about 1 in 20000 pregnancies (half following a hydatidiform mole, the other half after abortion or childbirth) and very rarely arises as an ovarian germ cell tumour usually produces human chorionic gonadotrophin, as a marker. Like the endodermal sinus tumour, it may also occur in young women, is highly malignant and chemosensitive. The progress of both tumours and the success of therapy can be judged by measurement of the appropriate tumour marker.

    Oestrogens produced by granulosa-theca cell tumours and androgens secreted by arrhenoblastomas (tubular androblastomas) can also be viewed as tumour markers.

    There is also increasing interest in the use of CA 125 (carcinoma antigen 125) as a tumour marker for the efficacy of chemotherapy in ovarian cancer. The level of CA 125 in serum is elevated in 80% of women with macroscopic ovarian cancer; the level rises with progression and falls with treatment to give a sensitivity and specificity of 80–90%.

A 30-year-old divorced computer programmer was admitted as an emergency under the physicians with a pyrexia of 39.5°C. Apart from general malaise, fever and night sweats she complained of frequency, slight dysuria, and intermittent pain in her lower abdomen. Two months earlier she had requested removal of a Dalkon shield intrauterine contraceptive device (IUCD), which had been in situ for 5 years, both because she no longer required contraception, but also because she had experienced some intermenstrual bleeding. She had not had intercourse since this time and her menstrual cycle had become regular with 4–5 days bleeding every 28–31 days after the device had been removed. She had otherwise been well and had not previously had any serious illness or operation. Her only pregnancy 7 years before had resulted in a normal delivery. Despite a thorough examination and detailed investigation, including an MSU, no specific cause for her swinging pyrexia could be identified. She was given an empirical 7-day course of cotrimoxazole and rapidly became apyrexial. She remained well for 2 months after this, but was subsequently readmitted complaining of a severe stabbing pain in both iliac fossae especially the left. She again complained of dysuria and frequency. She had not had intercourse, nor missed any periods since her previous admission. Her last period had been normal and had occurred 10 days earlier, but she had experienced slight intermenstrual bleeding during the 2 days prior to admission.

General examination confirmed a temperature of 39°C and a pulse rate of 120 beats/minute. There was no other abnormality on general examination, nor on examination of her respiratory or cardiovascular systems. Her abdomen was not distended, but she was extremely tender over her lower abdomen especially on the left side. A mass of approximately 8–10 cm diameter, apparently arising from the pelvis, could be palpated in the left iliac fossa. There was marked guarding and rebound tenderness in this area. Her bowel sounds were normal. Pelvic examination confirmed a left adnexal mass approximately equivalent in size to a grapefruit. The uterus was bulky, anteverted and displaced to the right by the mass. There was generalised pelvic tenderness most marked on the left side, but minimal excitation pain on moving the cervix. The right adnexum was not palpable. The following results were obtained: Hb 10.6 g/dl, WCC 14.8 x 10^{9}fl, ESR 76 mm/h; film 80% of polymorphs, 20% lymphocytes; MSU — *Escherichia coli*>10^5 organisms/ml.

A diagnosis of a pyosalpinx or tubo-ovarian abscess and a urinary tract infection was made and treatment with cephradine and metronidazole was commenced. After 36 hours her temperature was settling, but her pain persisted and the mass appeared to be enlarging. It was therefore decided to perform a laparotomy. This revealed a thick-walled tubo-ovarian mass of about 10 cm diameter, which was densely adherent to the posterior aspect of the broad ligament, sigmoid colon and pelvic sidewall. The uterus and right ovary and tube were normal. Histological examination of the tubo-ovarian abscess was reported as showing: '... an abscess filled with necrotic debris and pus which include large numbers of sulphur

granules. These are made up by colonies of filamentous bacteria ...'
There are no epithelioid granulomata and no areas of caseous
necrosis. There is no evidence of malignancy'.

1. What is the cause of this abscess?
2. How would you treat her?
3. What contraceptive advice would you give?

1. This patient has a tubo-ovarian abscess due to actinomycosis. This is probably related to the intrauterine device which she had been using until 2 months before her admission to hospital. The contraceptive effect of both inert and copper IUCDs is thought to be due to a sterile inflammatory reaction to a foreign body within the uterine cavity. Women wearing an IUCD are, however, 3–6 times more likely to develop sexually transmitted pelvic inflammatory disease (PID). The overall incidence of salpingitis in IUCD users is 1–2.5% but has been reported to be as high as 7% in populations prone to PID. A recent study has, however, suggested an inflammatory reaction in the fallopian tubes of just over a half of women wearing an IUCD. Although neither Gram positive nor Gram negative organisms have been detected in these patients, the possibility of infection due to *Chlamydia trachomatis*, *Mycoplasma hominis* and *T-mycoplasma* cannot be excluded.

   Pelvic infection due to actinomycosis is rare. The organism *Actinomycosis israeli* is a pleomorphic rod-shaped, Gram positive anaerobic bacterium which grows in tissues as granules. In draining pus, these granules measure 1–2 cm in diameter and are white or yellow in colour — so-called 'sulphur granules'. Microscopically, these are composed of a filamentous form of the bacterium and resemble fungal mycelia.

   Actinomycosis israeli can be detected in the lower genital tract by routine cervical cytology, but rarely causes infection in the absence of a foreign body. Actinomyces-like structures have been reported in the smears of up to 10% of IUCD wearers and a relationship with duration of use has been suggested. Female genital infection due to the organism is, however, rare and until 1970 only 200 cases had been reported in the world literature. Whether the recent increase in the incidence of this infection is due to increased awareness of the disease or increased use of the IUCD is not clear.

2. There are no specific features that distinguish pelvic actinomycosis from other forms of PID. It should, however, be suspected whenever PID is diagnosed in association with an IUCD. A vague systemic illness, similar to that experienced by this patient, may precede the acute onset of pelvic signs and symptoms. The presence of a unilateral pelvic mass is particularly suspicious. Conservative management of acute pelvic sepsis, or a pyosalpinx, using antibiotic therapy is usual. A poor clinical response following therapy with ampicillin or cephradine and metronidazole, as occurred in this case, is suggestive of actinomycosis and justifies a laparotomy.

   Excision of the infected tissues is appropriate and should be followed by prolonged antibiotic therapy for between 6 months and 2 years. Penicillin or tetracycline are the antibiotics of choice. For the first 7–10 days after surgery, metronidazole therapy should be maintained to eradicate any associated anaerobic bacteria.

3. This patient should be advised never to use an IUCD again.

An 80-year-old widow was referred to the gynaecology clinic complaining of vulval pruritis, soreness and swelling for 2 months. She was also troubled by a vaginal discharge and thought that this was probably the cause of her discomfort. Her periods had stopped when she was about 50 years of age and there was no history of postmenopausal bleeding. She had some frequency and urgency of micturition with occasional stress incontinence. She was also chronically constipated. Her general health was very good and she lived with 1 of her 5 children. Her past history included a prolapse repair at the age of 34 and an operation on her varicose veins some years later. She was not taking any medication.

On general examination she was a fit, sprightly lady who was not overweight. Her blood pressure was 140/90 mmHg and there was no abnormality of her cardiovascular or respiratory systems. Her breasts were atrophic, as were her vulva and vagina. The skin overlying the labia minora and majora was white in colour, in places it appeared thin and in others it was thickened. There were also signs of recent scratching, but no ulceration. She had a very small rectocoele and minimal cystocoele. There was no demonstrable stress incontinence, nor any obvious vaginal discharge. Her cervix appeared to have been amputated, probably at the time of the repair operation. The uterus was small, axial and mobile and there were no adnexal masses.

1. What condition is this woman suffering from?
2. What investigations would you perform to confirm this?
3. Classify the various appearances which this type of lesion can have.

1. This woman has a vulval dystrophy.

2. The only way in which this can be confirmed absolutely is to take a biopsy and obtain a histological diagnosis. However, taking a biopsy has the disadvantage that the area of excision may be slow to heal, and may even develop into a chronic ulcer. With experience, the diagnosis can be made clinically, thus avoiding the risks of biopsy. However, if the decision is made not to take a biopsy, it is essential to scan the vulval area very closely for any signs of malignancy. These include nodular or markedly thickened areas, ulceration, bleeding, and any sudden change in pigmentation. Should any of these occur, biopsy becomes mandatory. If biopsy is not performed, close follow-up is essential, with visual checks being made initially every 3 months; if there are no worrying signs after a year, follow-up visits can be decreased to 6 monthly.

3. Dystrophies of the vulva are chronic disorders of epithelial growth that result in alterations of the surface appearance and architecture. The changes seen may be localised or diffuse, hypotrophic or hypertrophic, and the skin may appear red where it is hypotrophic (thin, exposing the underlying blood vessels), or white where it is hypertrophic (thickened and opaque). There are essentially two forms: 'lichen sclerosus (et atrophicus)', where the skin is thinned and 'leukoplakia', where the skin is thickened. The two lesions may occur together forming a 'mixed dystrophy'.

   Lichen sclerosus is a lesion which usually affects postmenopausal women, but may occur in children or young adults. Its aetiology is unknown. The cardinal symptom is pruritis, but vulval soreness may also occur. Its appearance is variable. The skin usually looks thin, dry and 'parchment like' but fissures and ecchymoses may occur. As the lesion progresses, the labia minora and the clitoris and introitus shrink, producing the appearance of so-called 'kraurosis vulvae'. Microscopy reveals epithelial thinning, with loss of epithelial folds (rete ridges). The underlying dermis has an acellular appearance and frequently contains an inflammatory infiltrate at its lower margin.

   Hyperplastic dystrophy usually occurs in a younger age group (20–50 years). There may be a history of 'contact' irritation due to soap, deodorants or to persistent vulval moisture secondary to tight clothing and nylon underwear. Pruritis is the major symptom. It leads to scratching and this may be the factor inducing hyperplastic change. Vulval examination usually reveals thick white patches of variable size surrounded by red inflamed skin which may be excoriated from uncontrolled scratching. The microscopic appearance is characterised by thickening of the epithelium (hyperplasia) and keratin layer (hyperkeratosis). There is also widening of the epithelial rete ridges (acanthosis), retention of nuclear material in the keratin layer (parakeratosis) and chronic inflammation within the dermis. Leukoplakia is a term that has in the past been used both to describe 'white' skin and as a histological 'diagnosis' for certain hyperplastic lesions. Because of the confusion this term has caused, it is best avoided.

   Hyperplastic dystrophy can usually be eradicated if the scratch-itch cycle is broken with a course of mild corticosteroid cream, and precipitating factors are subsequently avoided. Lichen sclerosus frequently responds to oestrogen creams, combined if necessary with a mild topical steroid, for example 1% hydrocortisone cream or ointment. If this fails, topical 2% testosterone propionate two or three times daily for 4 weeks and thereafter twice weekly has been reported to be effective. Side effects of this latter therapy include clitoral enlargement and increased libido, but these seldom necessitate stopping treatment.

Biopsy in suspicious cases is necessary not only to make a diagnosis but also to exclude cellular atypia (dysplasia) or vulval intraepithelial neoplasia (VIN). This is very rare with lichen sclerosus, but occurs in up to 5% of hyperplastic lesions. Progression from mild vulval dysplasia (VIN I) to severe dysplasia or carcinoma in situ (VIN III) has not been demonstrated as clearly as it has for cervical dysplasia (cervical intraepithelial neoplasia CIN). These lesions should therefore be treated conservatively when they are observed in association with vulval dystrophies. Stopping the itching and the causal agent(s) may be all that is necessary. If there is an area of carcinoma in situ (intraepithelial carcinoma or VIN III) local excision is indicated. Because of the risk of malignant transformation, patients with vulval dystrophy should always be seen every 6 months. Primary vulval carcinoma in situ (VIN III) usually occurs in young women (median age between 30 to 40). Pruritis, pain and bleeding are the commonest symptoms. The lesions may be pink, white, red or brown and are often slightly elevated. Diagnosis can only be made by biopsy. Therapy is surgical with wide excision of affected areas or simple vulvectomy if necessary. Laser therapy to affected areas, or local application of the cytotoxic agent 5-fluorouracil (5-FU) have also been used with reported success.

Extramammary Paget's disease occurs in older women and produces moist reddish lesions. It may be associated with an underlying adenocarcinoma. Biopsy reveals pathognomonic large cells with clear vacuolated cytoplasm (Paget cells). Wide local excision or vulvectomy are indicated.

Biopsy in this patient revealed lichen sclerosus (et atrophicus) with hyperplastic areas. In view of her complaint of a vaginal discharge, a vault smear and high vaginal and vulval swabs were taken. These were normal. A midstream urine specimen was also cultured to exclude a urinary tract infection. Because of her postmenopausal bleeding, a diagnostic endometrial curettage was performed at the time of the vulval biopsy. This was also normal. Application of dienoestrol and 1% hydrocortisone creams on alternate days proved effective in alleviating her symptoms.

Gynaecology 30

A frail 90-year-old widow attended the gynaecology clinic complaining that she had noticed a blood stain on her underwear on several occasions over the previous 3–4 weeks. During this time she had also experienced intermittent frequency and dysuria. Her periods had stopped at the age of 52 years and she had not experienced any vaginal bleeding until the present episode. Her appetite had become poor, but her weight was constant. She had been treated with steroids (prednisolone 5 mg b.d) during the preceding month for polymyalgia of uncertain cause. She was not taking any other medication and had never suffered any major illness throughout her long life. She had three children, all of whom had been born normally. On examination she was remarkably 'well preserved' for her age. She was not overweight and her blood pressure was 150/100 mmHg. Apart from a slight clinical increase in cardiac size, there was no other abnormality of her respiratory or cardiovascular systems. Her breasts and abdomen were normal, apart from a palpable bladder. Vulval examination revealed an ulcerated tumour of approximately 3 cm diameter arising on the right side of the clitoris. The vagina was atrophic but otherwise normal. Her cervix and uterus were also atrophic but were mobile. There were no adnexal masses. Rectal examination was normal and there did not appear to be any palpable inguinal lymph nodes.

1. What is the likely diagnosis and how would you confirm this?
2. What is the likely histology of this lesion? Stage the tumour.
3. What treatment would you advise?
4. What is the prognosis following this treatment?

1. Biopsy of this old lady's vulval lesion showed that she had a stage II squamous cell carcinoma.

   Carcinoma of the vulva usually occurs in postmenopausal women after the age of 60 years. It accounts for approximately 5% of gynaecological malignancies and is the fourth most common primary pelvic cancer. Squamous cell carcinoma accounts for 90% of cases of vulval malignancy and sarcoma 5%. The remaining 5% include: adenocarcinoma (usually of Bartholin's glands or in association with Paget's disease), basal cell carcinoma and lymphoma.

   Seventy per cent of squamous carcinomas are labial and 15% are clitoral; the remainder arise elsewhere on the perineum.

2. Squamous cell carcinoma of the vulva is a slow-growing tumour which spreads directly to involve the vagina, urethra, anus and, in neglected cases, the underlying pubic bones. The perineal lymphatics form an extensive plexus which drain in sequence to the superficial and then deep inguinal nodes, and subsequently to femoral, iliac and para-aortic nodes. The cancer is staged by clinical criteria. In stage I and II the tumour is confined to the vulva and there is no evidence of inguinal node involvement. In stage I the diameter of the tumour is less then 2 cm and in stage II it is more than 2 cm. Stage III disease involves the vagina, urethra, perineum, anus or inguinal nodes. Stage IV involves the rectum, upper urethra, bladder, pelvic bones or distant metastases.

3. Once the diagnosis has been established, a chest X-ray and intravenous urogram, electrocardiogram, full blood count, blood urea, blood glucose, midstream urine and cervical smear should be obtained and cystoscopy and proctoscopy performed at the time of examination under anaesthesia prior to surgery. The standard procedure is a radical vulvectomy. This involves excision of the entire vulval skin and bilateral inguinal lymphadenectomy. The deepest node in the femoral canal (Cloquet's node) may be submitted to frozen section and, if positive, a deep pelvic node dissection may be performed to remove the external iliac, obturator and hypogastric nodes. The pelvic nodes are virtually never involved when Cloquet's node is negative.

   Tumour size is not a good guide to lymph node involvement, as approximately 10% of stage I tumours have metastases in the inguinal nodes.

   Because vulvectomy entails extensive skin loss, the operation is frequently complicated by wound breakdown and healing by granulation is not uncommon. Appropriate 'relieving' incisions can reduce skin tension and reduce wound necrosis. Because vulval skin is extremely radiosensitive, direct radiotherapy cannot be used to treat this tumour. External beam therapy may, however, be used to irradiate the pelvic nodes. Local recurrences, which cannot be removed surgically, have also been treated by local implantation of radium needles.

4. The 5-year survival of tumours confined to the vulva is 85%. This falls to 50% if the superficial inguinal nodes are involved and less than 15% with spread to the deep nodes.

Gynaecology 31

A 40-year-old housewife with two children aged 14 and 17 years was referred for a gynaecological opinion because she had experienced 6 months amenorrhoea. Shortly after the birth of her second child she had started taking a combined oral contraceptive pill. This suited her well and produced regular 3-day withdrawal bleeds every 28 days. She had reluctantly abandoned this method of contraception 6 months earlier on the advice of her family doctor. As she was a non-smoker and wanted to continue with an oral preparation, he had prescribed a progestogen-only pill containing 300 μg of ethynodiol diacetate. Initially she was very happy with this method and was pleased that she did not menstruate. After three missed periods, however, she became increasingly anxious about the possibility of an unwanted pregnancy. There was no other gynaecological complaint and repeated pregnancy tests were negative. She had deliberately lost 3 kg in weight over the previous 2 months, but her appetite and general health were good. She had not noted any secretion from her breasts, nor any change in her vision. She was not taking any other drugs and had never had any major illness or operation.

On examination she appeared to be a fit healthy woman. Her weight was 59.6 kg and her height 154 cm. There was no abnormality on general examination, nor on examination of her breasts or abdomen. Her blood pressure was 130/80 mmHg. Her vulva, vagina and cervix were of normal appearance and pelvic examination revealed a small, mobile, anteverted uterus with no adnexal masses. Her urine was normal on routine testing.

1. Comment on the contraceptive advice that this patient received from her doctor.
2. What investigations would you perform?
3. Assuming these all are normal — can you explain her amenorrhoea?
4. List the main indications for prescribing progestogen-only oral contraceptives.

1. The major cause of the excess mortality observed in users of combined oral contraceptive preparations is cardiovascular disease, i.e. myocardial infarction, cerebrovascular accidents, hypertension and thromboembolic disease. The incidence of these complications is age related, with approximately a 3-fold increase in risk in women who are in their late thirties. The risk is, however, much higher (5- to 7-fold) in women of this age who smoke or are markedly overweight. This patient should have been counselled about these risks when she was in her mid-thirties, and encouraged to consider another method of contraception. Her family doctor had, indeed, done this, but despite his advice she had remained adamant that she wished to continue with the combined pill and he had, therefore, quite reasonably, continued to prescribe it for her. She eventually relented and accepted his advice when she reached the age of 40. The fact that she is a non-smoker was relevant to the decision to allow her to continue on a combined oral contraceptive in her late thirties. It should not, however, have been of any importance in deciding whether to prescribe the progestogen-only pill for her. Although the progestogen component of combined oral contraceptive preparations is important in the aetiology of arterial vascular disease associated with the pill, use of progestogen-only preparations has not been shown to be associated with cardiovascular disease at any age.

2. Her secondary amenorrhoea probably resulted from her use of progestogen as a contraceptive. She should either have stopped taking it or have been fully investigated. She was not at all keen to stop the pill as she felt perfectly well while taking it and, once reassured that she was not pregnant, was quite happy not to be troubled by periods. The following hormone measurements were therefore performed: follicle stimulating and luteinising hormones, prolactin, testosterone, and free thyroxine index. These investigations and a full blood count and plasma glucose were all normal and she was therefore allowed to continue with her chosen contraceptive method.

   The main effect of the progestogen-only pill is to produce changes in the endocervical secretions which render these relatively hostile to sperm. It also causes some disruption of endometrial development. In nearly three-quarters of women who take these preparations, there is also some disruption of ovulation and/or the function of the corpus luteum.

3. Approximately a half of all women using this method experience either a delay in ovulation (causing prolonged menstrual cycles) or shortening of the luteal phase, resulting in a shorter interval between periods. In about a third of women taking this type of pill, ovulation may be inhibited entirely for two or more months leading to oligomenorrhoea — or more rarely, amenorrhoea (as in this case). There is therefore a paradox, in that the women who, because of missed periods, fear that they may be pregnant through failure of the method are probably those deriving the greatest contraceptive benefit from it.

4. The progestogen-only pill is suitable for any woman who is prepared to accept the risk of an unwanted pregnancy (3 per 100 women years, i.e. 3%) and the relatively high incidence of menstrual irregularity associated with the method (approximately 60–70%). It is also particularly useful for lactating women as it has no significant effect on milk quality or quantity and less than one-thousandth of the ingested dose is secreted in the milk. In addition, its contraceptive effect is virtually 100% in these women. It is generally advised for women with medical diseases in which the oestrogen component of the combined pill is best avoided, e.g. diabetes, hypertension, cardiac disease, etc. It is, however, important to be aware that, although the progestogen-only preparations have never been shown to produce any significant change in coagulation function, or to be associated with thromboembolic disease, they are nonetheless considered to be contraindicated by the manufacturers in patients with a past history of this condition.

Gynaecology 32

A 43-year-old married Indian laboratory assistant was admitted as an emergency with a history of heavy vaginal bleeding for 4 days. The blood loss had been so heavy that she was having to use babies' disposable nappies rather than sanitary towels. On the day of admission she had passed several large blood clots and this had been associated with colicky suprapubic pains. Her last menstrual period had occurred 4 months earlier and she had not experienced any other bleeding during this time. She admitted to frequent hot flushes, but had not had any treatment for these. During the preceding 3 years her menstrual cycle had been totally unpredictable with episodes of amenorrhoea lasting for between 6 weeks and 6 months. The bleeding lasted for between 8 and 15 days and had been especially heavy when the duration of amenorrhoea was prolonged. A diagnostic curettage performed approximately 6 weeks before her last period had shown normal proliferative endometrium. There was no history of intermenstrual nor postcoital bleeding, nor any other gynaecological problem. She had been sterilised (by tubal ligation) 14 years earlier after delivery of her sixth child. All six children had been born normally. She had also had 2 spontaneous first trimester abortions. There was no other relevant past medical or family history.

On examination she was of short stature (152 cm) and obese (72 kg). She looked slightly pale, but was otherwise healthy. There was no abnormality on general or abdominal examination. Pelvic examination revealed a normal vulva, vagina and cervix. The bleeding, which was coming through the cervix, was not unduly heavy. Her uterus was bulky, regular in outline, anteverted and mobile. There were no adnexal masses, nor any pelvic tenderness. Routine urine analysis was normal. Her haemoglobin was 10.1 g/dl with a normocytic blood film.

1. What is the most likely diagnosis?
2. How would you confirm this?
3. What treatment would you advise?
4. What is the relevance of her sterilisation?

1. Irregular uterine bleeding at any time during the reproductive phase of a woman's life may be due to an organic cause, or may be dysfunctional in origin, i.e. due to a disorder of the hypothalamo-pituitary-ovarian axis. Strictly speaking this latter diagnosis cannot be made without excluding organic pathology. Any woman in her late thirties or early forties who experiences irregular menstruation that is heavy or prolonged, should therefore have a diagnostic endometrial curettage to exclude intrauterine malignancy, adenomatous hyperplasia, a submucous fibroid polyp, or benign endometrial polyps. Endometrial sampling, which can often be done as an outpatient procedure using suction curettage, not only excludes intrauterine pathology, but may also provide a diagnosis when the bleeding is dysfunctional. In some centres, endoscopic examination of the endometrial cavity, i.e. hysteroscopy, is also performed.

2. Although this patient was only in her early forties, her history of hot flushes suggests that she is perimenopausal and this is the most likely cause of her irregular bleeding. When ovarian responsiveness to the pituitary gonadotrophins is reduced, tonic elevation of follicle-stimulating hormone (FSH) occurs. This causes continuous secretion of oestradiol by the ovaries in amounts which are sufficient to produce endometrial proliferation, but which fail to stimulate ovulation (either because of ovarian unresponsiveness, or a failure to 'trigger' the release of luteinising hormone release factor from the hypothalamus). The net result is prolonged unopposed oestrogen stimulation of the endometrium. This causes the stroma to become thickened and compact; the endometrial glands to increase in number and length and then to become cystic. Eventually the endometrium outgrows its blood supply and sloughs, frequently resulting in profound menorrhagia. A diagnostic curettage in this patient confirmed the diagnosis of 'cystic endometrial hyperplasia'.

   This pattern of menstrual irregularity, which has been termed 'metropathia haemorrhagica', also occurs at the time of puberty when the cyclic hormonal interactions are not fully established.

3. This patient should be treated initially with oral progestogens, e.g. norethisterone 5 mg t.i.d., medroxy-progesterone 10 mg t.i.d., or dydrogesterone 10 mg t.i.d. for 10 days. This will produce secretory changes in the endometrium and will induce a withdrawal bleed when it is stopped (so-called 'medical curettage'). Thereafter a lower dose of progestogen can be given on a cyclical basis for 12 days from day 14 to day 25 of the menstrual cycle. It is worth continuing this therapy for several months when the menopause is considered imminent. Because of the superior cycle control that can be achieved with oestrogen-progestogen preparations, some authorities advocate these in preference to progestogens alone. This practice has, however, been criticised because it is known that the risk of arterial vascular disease increases substantially in older women using the combined oral contraceptive pill. This argument is, however, probably spurious as it is now recognised that the risk of arterial disease in women treated with these preparations is related to the effect of the progestogen acting on the oestrogen-primed

environment rather than to the oestrogen itself. If prolonged progestogen therapy is likely to be necessary, then it may be better to perform a hysterectomy and this is often in any case more acceptable to the patient. Residual ovarian function should be conserved in these women.

4. The fact that this patient had previously had a sterilisation is not relevant to her menstrual problem.

The wife of a soldier in the Saudi Arabian National Guard was referred for investigation because of recurrent miscarriage. She was 29 years old and had a son aged 6, whose pregnancy and delivery at term had been entirely normal. Her subsequent 3 pregnancies had, however, ended in miscarriage at 8, 10 and 9 weeks gestation respectively, the last a year before referral. In each case the miscarriage had been preceded by slight vaginal bleeding for 3–4 days, but despite rest in bed, the bleeding had become heavier, lower abdominal cramps had developed and abortion had followed. Evacuation of retained products of conception had been performed after each miscarriage. For approximately 18 months she had experienced irregular periods at intervals of 4–7 weeks and clomiphene had been prescribed to achieve regular ovulation. She had started the treatment again after the latest miscarriage. Her periods occurred approximately every 28 days on this therapy. She had no other gynaecological complaints. Six months earlier she had sought the opinion of a private gynaecologist while on holiday in the United Kingdom. The only investigation performed was a laparoscopy and hydrotubation. This apparently revealed a normal uterus, ovaries and fallopian tubes and she had been reassured that there was no apparent cause for her miscarriages. Her general health was good and there was no relevant past medical, family or social history. On general examination she appeared to be a fit young woman. There was no abnormality of her breasts or abdomen. Pelvic examination was also entirely normal.

1. List the causes of miscarriage in the first trimester of pregnancy.
2. Comment on the role of laparoscopy in the investigation of habitual miscarriage.
3. What other investigations would you perform?
4. Assuming these are normal how would you manage her next pregnancy?

1. Approximately 60–80% of spontaneous first trimester miscarriages result from an abnormality of the conceptus. This may be either a congenital abnormality of the fetus, or an implantation defect. The former commonly include chromosomal disorders such as trisomy, triploidy and Turner's syndrome. These chromosomal anomalies are more likely to cause recurrent miscarriage than abnormalities of implantation, especially in older couples or those where one partner has a chromosomal defect, such as a balanced translocation.

   The remaining causes of miscarriage in early pregnancy are of maternal origin. These include medical disorders such as hypothyroidism, diabetes mellitus and renal disease. Chronic maternal infection may also be a cause of abortion. For example, syphilis and *Listeria monocytogenes* almost certainly cause recurrent miscarriage. Infection with the T-strain mycoplasmas such as *Ureaplasma urealyticum* has also been implicated as a cause of miscarriage. Viruses such as *cytomegalovirus* (CMV) and *Herpes simplex* and protozoa such as *Toxoplasma gondii* cause miscarriage on a 'one off' basis, but because immunity usually develops after the initial infection, are rarely if ever a cause of recurrent miscarriage. Occasionally, the parasite causing toxoplasma can persist in the blood for up to 2 years and thus cause repeated miscarriage during this time, although even if the mother has active infection only about 50% of fetuses become infected. Other maternal causes of abortion include acute infections which cause a high fever, such as influenza, pyelonephritis, etc., ingestion of noxious chemicals or cytotoxic agents, and anomalies of the uterus, both acquired — e.g. fibroids — and congenital, e.g. a bicornuate or subseptate uterus. Inadequate secretion of progesterone by the corpus luteum is also considered by some to be a maternal cause of miscarriage but this may be the result of deficient HCG production by a failing conceptus. There is also some evidence that failure of maternal recognition of paternal antigens carried by the fetus, with failure to produce the so-called 'blocking antibody' may also lead to miscarriage. (Cervical incompetence does not appear to cause abortion during the first trimester of pregnancy.)

   Finally, it must be borne in mind that a woman who is anxious to become pregnant, but has a prolonged (5–8 week) menstrual cycle, may think she has had several miscarriages when she has never ever been pregnant.

   Studies in which conception has been confirmed by measuring b-subunit HCG in maternal plasma, have shown that nearly 50% of pregnancies fail before they are diagnosed clinically. Approximately 15% of recognised pregnancies fail. In practice, the cause of miscarriage in most individual cases remains unknown.

2. Laparoscopy has no real place in the investigation of miscarriage. It would, of course, enable a major uterine anomaly to be recognised, but this is an unlikely cause of miscarriage in this patient who had previously had a normal full-term delivery. Furthermore, any gross abnormality in the shape of her uterine cavity would probably have been recognised during evacuation of retained products of conception which had been performed on three occasions.

3. Hysterosalpingography (HSG) is a simpler procedure and is of greater value than laparoscopy for excluding a congenital or acquired uterine anomaly. It may also be of value for assessing cervical incompetence in women with a history of recurrent midtrimester miscarriage. Appropriate investigation in this case would include: chromosome analysis of both partners; thyroid function tests; a glucose tolerance test; routine analysis and culture of a midstream uterine specimen; a blood urea estimation; a routine blood count; treponemal serology; a cervical swab cultured to exclude *Listeria monocytogenes*; testing for *Toxoplasma* IGM antibody titre; an HSG.

4. If these investigations are normal, then there are few specific measures that can be taken. These couples are usually advised to avoid intercourse during the first trimester and the women to avoid heavy physical exertion, although neither activity has ever been shown to precipitate miscarriage. Progestogen therapy, given on an empirical basis, is no longer considered to be of value. Serial measurement of maternal plasma progesterone concentrations, 2 or 3 times a week, may be of help in assessing corpus luteum function. If these are found to be low then treatment with HCG 6000 units 2 or 3 times weekly until approximately the 14th week of pregnancy, appears logical. However, it remains to be demonstrated in a randomised double-blind trial that such therapy is truly effective. Emotional support and 'tender loving care' are important for all pregnant women and especially for those who have a history of habitual abortion. Demonstrating normal fetal development by regular ultrasound scans from 8 weeks gestation onwards often has a markedly beneficial psychological effect.

Gynaecology 34

A 56-year-old Department of Health training officer was referred to the gynaecology clinic by her GP for retrieval of a 'lost' IUCD. She had been having irregular and quite heavy periods for the previous 18 months and, assuming that she was now approaching the menopause and therefore unlikely to conceive, asked for her IUCD to be removed. The IUCD strings had been missing for most of the 15 years it had been in situ, but a plain X-ray 5 years earlier and an ultrasound scan 2 years after that confirmed the intrauterine presence of the IUCD. With the exception of persistent hot flushes and regular night sweats, she had no symptoms. She was a non-smoker and a cervical smear 3 years previously had been reported as normal.

Examination revealed a healthy looking, rather overweight woman with no clinical evidence of anaemia. Her BP was 160/90 and there were no abdominal masses palpable. The vulva, vagina and cervix looked normal and the uterus was normal in size, anteverted and mobile. At the patient's request, no further attempts were made to remove the IUCD without anaesthetic and she was subsequently admitted so that it could be done under general anaesthesia. The IUCD, a Lippes loop, was easily retrieved after dilating the cervix, but there was more endometrium adherent to the IUCD than might usually have been expected and so a careful curettage was performed and bulky curettings obtained. The uterine cavity was 7 cm in length and there were no endocervical curettings. Histology showed the presence of poorly differentiated endometrial carcinoma.

1. The patient's first question after being told of the findings was whether the IUCD could have caused the malignancy. Could this have been so?
2. What features in the history are suggestive of endometrial cancer?
3. What are the next steps in the management of this case?

1. There is no evidence that IUCDs cause any form of cancer.

2. Endometrial carcinoma is usually associated with low parity, obesity, hypertension and a history of heavy prolonged periods of the sort usually associated with anovulation and unopposed oestrogen activity. The older the patient is at the menopause, the greater the risk of endometrial carcinoma.

3. This lady had a stage I, grade 3 endometrial carcinoma with tumour extending deeply into the myometrium. Treatment in this sort of case usually consists of hysterectomy/bilateral salpingo-oophorectomy and radiotherapy, but authorities are divided as to whether radiotherapy should precede or follow surgery because of the difficulty in assessing the exact extent of the disease preoperatively. Those who favour giving radiotherapy postoperatively do so on the basis that in the absence of deep myometrial involvement the incidence of lymph node metastases is relatively low and in view of its side effects the use of radiotherapy in such cases is not justified. Since the tumour in this particular case extended deeply into the myometrium, radiotherapy was given after surgery and consisted of both intravaginal radium and external irradiation of the pelvic field. Adjuvant progestogen therapy was not used because poorly differentiated tumours are less responsive than well differentiated ones.

Gynaecology 35

A 77-year-old nulliparous widow was referred to her local hospital because of a single episode of postmenopausal vaginal bleeding. She described the blood loss as 'watery and a little smelly — not like a real period'. Her past history included a Fothergill repair when she was 42 and a diagnostic curettage for postmenopausal bleeding when she was 56 years old: nothing abnormal was found.

She had never had a cervical smear and was otherwise in good health. Her only medication was a mild aperient, which she took as required.

Examination in the outpatient clinic was unremarkable, but in view of the history she was admitted for diagnostic curettage. This revealed a generalised atrophy of the vulva, vagina and cervix, a normal size uterus and no adnexal masses. A little pus was obtained from the uterine cavity but no curettings. The pus was sent for culture but failed to grow any organism.

She was seen three weeks later in the outpatient clinic. She reported that she was still bleeding small amounts each day. Her haemoglobin was 13.8 g/dl and chest X-ray was normal.

1. What are the possible causes of purulent uterine discharge in a patient such as this?
2. How should she be managed now?

1. A purulent discharge may be associated with long-standing atrophy and genital infection, but in a patient like this the most likely cause is an endometrial malignancy, despite the negative curettage.

2. Given the purulent discharge and postmenopausal bleeding, endometrial carcinoma must be highly likely. Since curettage had failed to reveal any intrauterine pathology, it was felt that hysterectomy was the only other way of establishing a diagnosis and so was performed in this case. The uterus was found to contain a well differentiated endometrial carcinoma (stage I grade 1) with no evidence of invasion into the myometrium. The ovaries were removed at the time and were clear of tumour.

   Although the value of adjuvant progestogen therapy in stage I disease has not been proved, it was felt that this patient might benefit and certainly would come to no harm from it. Nevertheless she declined further therapy on the grounds that, as a childless widow living in a residential home and 'without that much to look forward to' she had no fear of death. Spirited discussions on a number of occasions subsequently failed to shake her resolve, but she attended the outpatient clinic regularly over the next 18 months 'for want of something to do'. She died peacefully in her sleep 22 months after her hysterectomy.

Gynaecology 36

A 64-year-old widow with two children was referred to the gynaecological outpatient clinic by one of the consultant physicians in the hospital group. She had been under his care for the previous few months for the investigation of persistent numbness in her left leg and occasional chest pains. Her cardiovascular system had been thoroughly investigated and found to be normal, but chest X-ray showed a small right-sided hydrothorax. The numbness in her leg was attributed to lumbar vertebral disc degeneration.

When seen in the gynaecology clinic the patient complained only of a dragging sensation in the pelvis. This had gradually become worse and was exacerbated by long periods of standing; it was relieved by lying down. Her menopause had been 10 years earlier and there had been no postmenopausal bleeding.

Examination revealed a cheerful, rather obese lady who was able to lie flat without difficulty. Abdominal palpation was made difficult by her obesity, but there was no evidence of ascites or any abdominal mass. The vulva and vagina were normal, as was the cervix. There was a small cystocoele but minimal uterovaginal descent. The uterus was difficult to define bimanually, but there was a definite left-sided adnexal mass approximately 6–8 cm in diameter. Ultrasound scan showed a normal-size uterus with a solid left adnexal mass. Routine haemoglobin was 11.8 g/dl, ESR 8 mm/hour and electrolytes within normal limits. A repeat chest X-ray confirmed the right-sided hydrothorax, but no other abnormality and a bone scan showed no areas suggestive of secondary deposits.

1. What is the most likely diagnosis?
2. How would you manage the problem subsequently?
3. What is the outlook?

1. As a rough guide, the likelihood of ovarian masses proving to be malignant can be said to be about 50% in prepubertal and postmenopausal women and about 10% in women during their potentially reproductive years. This is largely because functional (benign) ovarian cysts are so common in the latter group. In this case, therefore, the patient was advised to undergo laparotomy in order to ascertain the nature of the mass.

2. After opening the abdomen through a midline incision the peritoneal cavity was found to contain a moderate volume of straw-coloured fluid. There was an 8 cm diameter freely mobile mass involving the left ovary, but the right ovary and uterus were normal, as were the liver, spleen, omentum and intestines. The ovarian mass was opened immediately after removal and found to be solid in nature with no haemorrhagic areas. It was assumed to be a benign fibroma and so the procedure was restricted to left oophorectomy, though it must be said that most authorities would recommend total hysterectomy and bilateral salpingo-oophorectomy at this age, or at least a frozen section, in case the mass was found to be malignant and because of the risk of a tumour arising in the remaining ovary. The mass was in fact demonstrated histologically to be a fibroma, confirming the diagnosis of Meig's syndrome.

3. Although between 3% and 5% of ovarian tumours are fibromas, less than 5% of these are associated with the classical Meig's syndrome. This is defined as consisting of any benign solid ovarian tumour (usually a fibroma), ascites, hydrothorax and, importantly, cure of the fluid collections following removal of the tumour. The outlook is excellent.

A 20-year-old nulliparous au pair was referred to the gynaecology outpatient clinic from the local family planning clinic where she had attended requesting contraceptive advice. Routine examination at the time had revealed the presence of a right-sided pelvic swelling and she was therefore advised to see a gynaecologist, even though she was asymptomatic.

Her menarche had been at the age of 14 years and her menstrual cycle was regular, the periods lasting 4 days every 28–30 days. She had no intermenstrual or postcoital bleeding, nor any dyspareunia and had not used any form of contraception in the past.

Examination revealed a normal healthy female with no mass palpable abdominally. Vaginal examination, however, revealed a 6–8 cm mass lying anteriorly and to the right of the retroverted uterus.

1. What is the most likely diagnosis?
2. How would you confirm it?
3. How should she be managed further?

1. The diagnosis of an ovarian cyst can be made in most cases on clinical examination with no further investigation required. If, however, there is any doubt an ultrasound scan can be performed, since pregnancy, fibroids, or even a full bladder can confound the diagnosis.

2. Assuming that the mass is genuinely ovarian, the most likely types of cyst in a woman of this age would be a simple follicular cyst, or a dermoid cyst. The fact that in this particular case the cyst was lying anterior to the uterus makes it more likely to be a dermoid. A plain abdominal X-ray showed the presence of teeth, confirming the diagnosis of a dermoid cyst.

3. The treatment for any cyst of this size is laparotomy and ovarian cystectomy, making every attempt to conserve as much ovary as possible since even the most distorted ovary is capable of quite remarkable regeneration. Although malignant change in a benign teratoma is rare, it is best to remove the cyst intact if possible. A careful dissection was performed in this case and a compressed piece of ovarian tissue conserved. Histology confirmed that the cyst was a benign dermoid.

Gynaecology 38

A 25-year-old married nurse had an emergency caesarean section performed for fetal distress associated with a placental abruption at 38 weeks gestation. The baby was delivered safely, but the postnatal recovery was complicated by puerperal pyrexia and a foul-smelling vaginal discharge.

She was next seen 3 years later in the gynaecology outpatient clinic complaining of infertility. She had started trying for a second child 6 months after her caesarean section, having relied on the sheath for contraception during this time. She was still married to the same husband, had remained in good health and menstruated regularly for 4 days out of every 28.

Nothing untoward was found on examination and a postcoital test on the 12th day of her cycle showed plentiful actively motile spermatozoa in a copious clear mucus. Serum prolactin was 258 mu/l, FSH 4.6 u/l, LH 6.0 u/l and thyroid function was normal. Her temperature chart was clearly biphasic and day 21 serum progesterone suggestive of ovulation (>40 nmol/l).

Diagnostic laparoscopy was therefore performed and revealed a normal uterus, right tube and ovary. The left tube, however, was bound down by adhesions to the back of the broad ligament and there was evidence of chronic sepsis and adhesions in the pouch of Douglas. The left ovary could not be seen. Methylene blue dye was injected through the cervix and passed easily through the right tube but not the left.

1. How significant is the finding of unilateral tubal blockage in this particular case?
2. What further investigation should be performed before embarking on treatment?
3. If the tubal blockage is responsible for this lady's secondary infertility, what can be done in the way of treatment?

1. The laparoscopic findings may not be totally conclusive, as in this case where only one tube appeared to be occluded; given the history one might expect both tubes to be affected. Failure to achieve tubal fill and spill of dye may be due to factors other than tubal occlusion — a poor seal at the cervix and an intrauterine septum being two possibilities. Tubal spasm has been postulated as a cause of apparent tubal blockage, but this is very hard to prove as an entity.

2. Hysterosalpingography should performed whenever the laparoscopic findings are not be totally conclusive. In this patient, the HSG revealed fill and spill from both tubes, albeit very sluggishly from the left tube. A 'smearing' effect was noted, consistent with the distortion of the anatomy caused by adhesions.

   The fact that tubal patency was proved in this case does not automatically mean that a conception will occur, since the motility and epithelial function of the tube may not be normal. There is also a not inconsiderable risk of ectopic pregnancy and this should be carefully explained to the patient.

3. If the patient is not prepared to wait for a pregnancy to occur spontaneously, there is an alternative, which is to bypass the fallopian tubes completely, recovering ova from the ovary under ultrasound or laparoscopic control and relying on extracorporeal fertilisation and reimplantation of the embryo. This procedure probably has a greater success rate where tubal blockage is the only reason for infertility, but has the major disadvantages of being expensive and offering only one chance of conception per treatment cycle.

   This lady chose in vitro fertilisation. After ovarian stimulation with gonadotrophins, four ova were collected under laparoscopic control. Two were successfully fertilised and reimplanted into the uterine cavity where one established and continued to term, when she delivered vaginally after a spontaneous labour.

Gynaecology 39

A 36-year-old mother of three was referred to the gynaecology clinic by her local family planning clinic with a covering letter explaining that the thread of a Copper 7 IUCD inserted at her 6-week postpartum visit 3 years earlier could no longer be felt or seen. The patient's husband had recently been given the all-clear following his vasectomy and she was therefore keen to have the IUCD removed.

On direct questioning the patient revealed that she had experienced sharp lower abdominal pain on insertion of the coil, but this had resolved with rest and she left the clinic after 1 hour's rest. There was no menstrual disturbance subsequently and she was certain that she had not lost the coil, even though the thread had not been palpable since her first postinsertion check-up. She mentioned that from time to time she suffered an intense pricking sensation around the anal region which her general practitioner had diagnosed as piles.

Examination in the clinic was normal, with no sign of the IUCD thread even after gently sounding the uterus with a barbed plastic thread retriever. Since the patient had just finished a normal period, a plain abdominal X-ray was taken and showed the presence of the coil in the pelvis. The patient was advised that it would be necessary to have the IUCD removed under general anaesthetic.

After anaesthesia had been administered the uterus was gently explored using a sound followed by a small polyp forceps. The coil was not found and therefore laparoscopy was performed: despite a good view of the pelvis, the IUCD could not be seen. Somewhat reluctantly laparotomy was carried out, but the IUCD could still not be found in the pelvis, nor was it in the omentum. On careful palpation, however, the coil was felt within the lumen of the ileum, approximately 20 cm from the ileocaecal junction. Further examination showed that this part of the ileum was firmly adherent to the rectum, with generalised thickening surrounding the point of adherence. Further dissection finally revealed the cross arm of the IUCD in the ileum with the tail and nylon thread in the rectum.

1. What is the significance of severe pain at the time of insertion of an IUCD?
2. Was there anything in the history that might have suggested that the coil was lying in a site other than the uterus?
3. How useful is abdominal X-ray in localising a 'lost' IUCD?
4. What is the role of laparoscopy in the location of lost copper coils?

1. The insertion of an IUCD is often accompanied by some discomfort, but this is rarely severe and should subside fairly quickly. When this is not the case, perforation should always be borne in mind. Uterine perforation is more common during postpartum insertions.

2. One should always suspect that perforation has occurred if the thread cannot be felt and the patient is certain it has not been expelled, though it is possible to lose an IUCD without noticing it. The pricking sensation reported by the patient may well have been due to a number of causes other than the IUCD thread, but since this symptom disappeared immediately after removal of the IUCD it must be assumed that it was due to the thread.

3. An abdominal X-ray will show the presence of a radio-opaque device in the pelvis, but is not always helpful in determining whether the device is intra- or extrauterine. Fitting another coil may help by identifying the uterine cavity. A pelvic ultrasound scan with a high resolution machine and experienced operator is probably more useful in this respect.

4. Most lost IUCDs can be removed by laparoscopy, but care should be taken with copper-covered devices because they are often covered with adhesions or in the omentum. Laparotomy should be performed unless one can be sure that laparoscopic removal will not cause untoward bleeding or damage.

Gynaecology 40

A 34-year-old married woman with three children became pregnant following a sheath failure. After much discussion, she and her husband consulted their general practitioner with a view to referral for termination of pregnancy, but before seeing the local gynaecologist she developed heavy vaginal bleeding with clots. She was seen again by the general practitioner who diagnosed a complete abortion and gave her an intramuscular injection of ergometrine 0.5 mg.

Two days later she developed further lower abdominal pain and began to bleed vaginally, again quite heavily. This time she was referred as an emergency to the local hospital, where an incomplete abortion was diagnosed and evacuation of retained products advised. At examination under anaesthetic the uterus was noted to be enlarged to a size approximately equivalent to the duration of amenorrhoea with the cervix sufficiently dilated to accept a 10 Hegar dilator. There were bilateral mobile adnexal masses, 5–6 cm and 8–10 cm diameter on the left and right sides respectively. A sponge-holding forceps was introduced into the uterine cavity and a copious amount of vesicular material obtained and sent for histological examination. This revealed large, poorly vascularised villi with proliferating trophoblast showing vacuolation. The appearances were those of a hydatidiform mole.

1. What are the bilateral adnexal masses and what should be done about them?
2. What are the next steps in the management of this patient?
3. How should she be followed up on a long-term basis?

1. The bilateral adnexal swellings are ovarian theca lutein cysts. They are caused by the high levels of HCG secreted by the trophoblast tumour acting on the ovaries to produce excessive luteinisation, which may take the form of lutein or follicular cysts. Nothing should be done about them because they nearly always regress spontaneously once the high levels of HCG produced by the trophoblast fall.

2. One of the cornerstones of treatment of hydatidiform moles is to ensure that the uterine cavity is completely empty and, for this reason, it was traditionally recommended that a further D & C be performed some 10–14 days after the initial removal of the mole. An alternative approach is to monitor the situation with serial ultrasound scans and HCG estimations. Prophylactic chemotherapy with methotrexate at the time of evacuation will reduce the number of cases requiring subsequent chemotherapy, but is probably unjustified because of the very small number of cases that would develop invasive disease.

3. Long-term follow-up is based on the early identification of any increase in HCG which would suggest that there is still hormone-secreting trophoblastic tumour present. It relies on the submisssion of regular urine samples for HCG estimation and, if the level is found to be increasing, serum HCG is estimated. Follow-up will range from 6 months to 2 years depending on the rate of fall of the urinary HCG. Pregnancy should be avoided during the follow-up period for the simple reason that it is impossible to differentiate the HCG secreted from a normal pregnancy from that produced by recurrent trophoblastic disease. Providing the HCG levels have remained normal for at least 12 and preferably 24 months (confirmed on serum assay), the patient can then be allowed to embark on a further pregnancy. Subsequent estimations of HCG 3 weeks and 3 months after any future pregnancy are advised because of the small increased risk of choriocarcinoma in such patients. Oestrogen or progesterone preparations for contraceptive or other purposes taken between the evacuation of the mole and the return of gonadotrophin values to normality appear to double the risk of invasive mole or choriocarcinoma requiring therapy and it is therefore suggested that these be avoided until HCG has become undetectable in serum.

Gynaecology 41

A 35-year-old housewife attended her local well woman clinic for a cervical smear. She had 2 children aged 8 years and 6 years; the second had been delivered by caesarean section because of placenta praevia. She then used the combined pill for contraception until her general practitioner advised her to stop because of her age and the fact that she smoked in excess of 20 cigarettes daily. Her husband then had a vasectomy and she stopped taking the pill as soon as he had had 2 negative sperm counts, which was 6 months before the current consultation.

The smear was reported as showing groups of moderately dyskaryotic cells present together with groups and fragments of elongated cells with hyperchromatic nuclei, the nature of which were uncertain. She was therefore referred to the local hospital where she was seen in the colposcopy clinic.

Using 10 times magnification, the entire transformation zone could be visualised as could the squamo-columnar junction. It was noted that at some points the columnar epithelium appeared to be more vascular than expected. There were distinct areas of punctation and mosaicism within the transformation zone and the entire area stained deeply white when 5% acetic acid was applied. Biopsies were taken from the most vascular part of the squamo-columnar junction and from the most abnormal area of the transformation zone. Haemostasis was secured using silver nitrate sticks gently pressed against the cervix.

The histology of the first biopsy showed adenocarcinoma in situ whilst the second revealed a moderate degree of dysplasia amounting to a CIN II.

There were also koilocytic atypia suggestive of wart virus infection.

1. How commonly might a combination of early cancers such as this occur in the same patient?
2. What is the significance of the presence of wart virus infection?
3. What is the correct management of this patient?

1. Adenocarcinoma in situ (AIS) of the cervix has been recognised for many years and at least one-third of cervical adenocarcinomas are associated with CIN of the squamous epithelium. Cervical adenocarcinoma is less common than the squamous type, with a reported incidence of between 5% and 10% of all cervical cancers, though it has recently been suggested that the incidence is rising. This increase may simply reflect better diagnostic methods, or it may be due to the more widespread use of oestrogen-containing preparations such as the pill. It may also share a common aetiology with the squamous carcinomas, i.e. the human papilloma virus.

2. It is now accepted that squamous carcinoma of the cervix does not occur in the absence of sexual activity. Evidence is accumulating that the human papilloma virus (particularly types 16 & 18), transmitted sexually, is implicated in the causation of cervical cancer, together with other possible contributory factors such as pregnancy at an early age, prolonged oral contraceptive usage and cigarette smoking. Any woman with genital warts, or a partner who has genital warts, should have cervical cytology performed as soon as the infection is diagnosed and again 1 year later.

3. Adenocarcinoma in situ, with or without squamous CIN, can theoretically be treated the same way as a squamous lesion alone. Unfortunately, it is often very difficult to visualise the epithelium of the endocervical canal sufficiently well to ensure that any local destructive therapy has been sufficient. Cone biopsy may offer a more reliable alternative, though in a woman who has completed her childbearing many authorities would advise hysterectomy with careful clinical follow-up and regular vault smears thereafter.

'She's got this terrible discharge', said the young mother, holding her 4-year-old daughter on her lap. 'It stains her underclothes and it must be hurting her because she cries whenever she passes her water. Our family doctor has given her all sorts of tablets and even the same cream she gave me when I had thrush but the discharge always comes back.'

On further questioning, it appeared that although there were two other girls in the family, both older, neither they nor their mother had any vaginal discharge or soreness. The 4-year-old had always been well and was the sort of child who rarely complained. The family lived in their own home and the mother always took care to wash all the children's underclothes separately from their other clothes, though they were done together in a washing machine. There was no family history of diabetes.

With the mother's help it was possible to make a simple examination of the little girl's vulva. This revealed a reddened and excoriated area with a small amount of discharge present around the labia minora.

1. What is the most likely cause of this discharge?
2. What other possible causes might give the same symptoms and signs?
3. What is the most effective treatment?

1. The commonest cause of vulvovaginitis in a girl of this age is a non-specific or mixed infection. The organisms responsible include *E. coli*, streptococci and staphylococci.

2. Similar symptoms and signs can be due to infection with pinworms, *trichomonas* and *monilia*. Infection secondary to the presence of a foreign body can also cause vulvovaginitis. The key in this particular case is the patient's age: foreign bodies, *trichomonas* and *monilia* tend to occur in older girls. Where there is any doubt, examination under anaesthetic should be performed. Furthermore, however unlikely it may appear, the possibility of sexual abuse must be borne in mind.

3. Local oestrogen therapy is the treatment of choice and works by lowering the vaginal pH, encouraging the growth of lactobacilli and inhibiting other organisms. Small amounts of the oestrogen cream should be applied gently to the labia and vaginal introitus, preferably by the child's mother, two or three times weekly until the discharge clears.

Gynaecology 43

A 55-year-old shop assistant complained that she was 'always wet down below'. This was not a recent problem, having begun shortly after the birth of her youngest child 27 years earlier, but since her menopause at the age of 51 the problem had become worse. She leaked small volumes of urine whenever she coughed or sneezed, but could hold on if she had to, provided that she sat still. There was no frequency during the daytime, but she had to get up at least four times each night to pass urine.

General examination was normal. Vaginal examination revealed a moderately atrophic lower genital tract with very little prolapse of the bladder neck. Even though her bladder was partially full at the time of the examination, there was no demonstrable urine loss. The cervix, uterus and adnexa were all normal.

1. What additional information would you like from the history?
2. Would you perform any special investigations and if so, why?
3. How likely is this to be genuine stress incontinence in the absence of prolapse and demonstrable incontinence?

1. The two most likely causes of intermittent urinary incontinence are genuine stress incontinence (GSI) and detrusor instability. The former usually occurs when the intra-abdominal pressure is greater than the intraurethral pressure, whilst the latter has a much more complex aetiology resulting in an inability to inhibit detrusor contraction. Patients with GSI generally present with incontinence related to anything that causes intra-abdominal pressure to exceed intraurethral pressure, i.e. coughing or sneezing; whereas those with detrusor instability can have any of a number of symptoms including frequency, nocturia, urgency and urge incontinence. In this case, therefore, the history of nocturia in what would otherwise sound like GSI needs further elucidation. Direct questioning revealed that the patient was used to taking several cups of tea each evening, and after advising her to take no drinks after 9pm her nocturia ceased.

2. Detrusor instability and GSI can, and often do, coexist in the same patient making both accurate diagnosis and, more importantly, appropriate treatment more difficult. In a case such as this (once the cause of the nocturia had been found) the diagnosis is quite clear and further investigation is unlikely to alter management. However, where the exact cause for the incontinence is unclear, cystometry should be performed to measure the detrusor pressure changes under different circumstances.

3. GSI is usually, but not invariably, associated with demonstrable bladder neck descent and will occur whenever the intraurethral pressure is decreased. It will occur in nulliparous women and when previous bladder neck surgery has been performed, as well as in young women following childbirth. In cases where no bladder neck descent is found, great care should be taken in making a diagnosis since surgery is unlikely to improve detrusor instability.

Gynaecology 44

A 15-year-old girl was brought to the outpatient clinic by her mother. The girl, slim and slightly small for her age, sat quietly while her mother did all the talking: 'Sorry to bother you doctor, but my daughter was 15 last month and she hasn't started her periods yet. My older daughter started hers when she was 13 and I seem to remember I started mine when I was about that age too. All the other girls in her class have started theirs and now she feels she is the odd one out. Do you think she might have a blockage somewhere?'

Having persuaded the girl to answer for herself, further questioning revealed that she had not noticed any abdominal pain or discomfort in her vagina and that she was more concerned about lack of breast development than absence of periods. She had a good appetite, got on well with her older sister and was happy at school.

On examination she was about 5 cm below average height for her age and about 6 kg underweight. There was early axillary and pubic hair growth and her breasts had started to enlarge. There were no abdominal masses palpable and gentle vaginal examination revealed a normal hymenal ring which just admitted the tip of a finger. A rectal examination confirmed the presence of a uterus.

1. What are the possible causes of primary amenorrhoea?
2. How would you establish a diagnosis?
3. How would you manage this particular case?

1. Possible causes of primary amenorrhoea include congenital abnormalities ranging from imperforate hymen to absence of the vagina, uterus or ovaries. Disorders of pituitary, thyroid, adrenal and ovarian function, sex chromosome abnormalities (XO, XX/XO, XY/XO) and end organ resistance (e.g. testicular feminization) must also be considered, together with eating disorders such as anorexia or bulimia and strenuous athletic activities beginning before and after puberty.

2. A careful history is naturally important in establishing a diagnosis, but in this particular situation the most useful starting point is physical examination — does the patient appear to be a normal postpubertal female? If she does, and especially if she gives a history of monthly abdominal pain or discomfort, then she should be examined vaginally to exclude an imperforate hymen and confirm the presence of the reproductive organs. It is always advisable to have the patient's mother and the clinic nurse present for this, even if the doctor is female.

   If the patient doesn't appear to have secondary sexual characteristics, diagnosis is more difficult. Chromosomal studies, serum FSH and LH, thyroid function tests and hand X-ray to determine bone age may all be necessary.

3. If there is no obvious cause for the primary amenorrhoea, such as in this case, reassurance alone is perfectly reasonable, together with advice about diet and the avoidance of extreme physical activity. A careful explanation of the basics of menstrual cycle control will greatly help and will serve as a useful baseline for discussing contraception at a later date. If the patient (or her mother) are still concerned, it may be worth performing a progestogen withdrawal test. The patient is given 5 mg of norethisterone 3 times daily for 3 days. A withdrawal bleed indicates that the reproductive system is functioning and the genital tract open. Oestrogen-containing preparations should not be used for this hormonal trial because they may inhibit the development of the hypothalamus and pituitary at a time when this is critical.

Gynaecology 45

A 29-year-old teacher and her 36-year-old husband, also a teacher, were referred by their general practitioner for investigation after they had been trying for a pregnancy for almost 4 years. She had never been pregnant and he had not fathered a child before. Both were in good health, were non-smokers and drank alcohol 'in moderation'.

Examination of both revealed no abnormality. Her serum prolactin, FSH/LH and thyroid function were normal and the temperature chart she had been keeping over the previous 6 months suggested ovulation was occurring. A postcoital test on the 12th day of her 28-day cycle revealed a copious clear mucus with long spinnbarkeit, but only a few sluggishly motile spermatozoa. A semen analysis was therefore requested and reported as containing 12 million spermatozoa/ml with 50% motility and 30% abnormal forms in a total volume of 3 ml. Two further tests at 3-weekly intervals and after 3 days of abstinence were similar. Although it now seemed clear that this couple's infertility was probably due to the male partner, a diagnostic laparoscopy was undertaken on the female and this confirmed the presence of a normal uterus, tubes and ovaries. After 6 unsuccessful attempts at artificial insemination with the husband's semen (AIH), GIFT was advised.

This was carried out 2 months later. Following the initial signs of pregnancy, including breast tenderness and nausea, to the couple's great disappointment, she began a period after 27 days. The period was lighter than normal and she continued to spot over the following week. She developed worsening right iliac fossa pain and was clinically tender on bimanual examination, which also suggested the presence of a 4 cm diameter mass on the right. This was confirmed on ultrasound scan together with the presence of free fluid in the pouch of Douglas.

1. What is GIFT?
2. What is the right adnexal mass?
3. How would you confirm the diagnosis?
4. How could this woman now achieve a pregnancy?

1. GIFT stands for gamete intrafallopian transfer. Up to four oocytes are collected from a deliberately overstimulated ovary and placed in a fine catheter which has already been loaded with about 50000 spermatozoa. Using laparoscopy, the gametes are then inserted into the fallopian tube through the fimbrial ends, using a fine plastic cannula. The overall success rate is variously estimated at about 30% and of these 15–20% will be ectopic pregnancies.

2. The right adnexal mass could be a persistent follicle, a corpus luteum cyst, or an ectopic pregnancy.

3. A positive monoclonal antibody beta-hCG pregnancy test would be highly suggestive of ectopic pregnancy, but laparoscopy would provide the definitive diagnosis.

4. This woman still has her left tube so GIFT could be tried once more. Alternatively, she could have 'full' in vitro fertilisation with the insertion of a number of fertilised and developing embryos into the uterine cavity.

Gynaecology 46

A 22-year-old woman, married with two children, was brought to the accident and emergency department late one night by her husband. They had been celebrating their fourth wedding anniversary at a local hostelry when she developed severe colicky right-sided abdominal pain. Since the hospital was only a short distance from the pub, they felt it would be easier to call in there rather than call out their GP.

On arrival in the A & E department she was in a stable condition, albeit somewhat the 'worse for wear' as a result of alcohol consumption. Her pulse was 90 and regular, her BP 120/80 and there was no clinical pallor. There was definite guarding over the right iliac fossa, but no mass was palpable. Vaginal examination revealed a small amount of bleeding from the cervix together with an IUCD thread. The uterus was normal-sized and mobile and, although there was definite tenderness in the right iliac fossa, there was no mass nor any cervical excitation tenderness. The patient confirmed that her last normal period had been two weeks earlier and that she often had mid-cycle bleeding.

In the absence of any strong diagnostic signs, a provisional diagnosis of mittelschmerz was made and the patient reassured. Admission to hospital for the night was offered in view of her inebriation, but she declined and was taken home by her husband.

Late the following evening she was again brought in to the A&E department this time by ambulance following a sudden exacerbation of her pain. She was clinically shocked, pale and peripherally vasoconstricted, her pulse was thready at 120 beats/minute and BP unrecordable. There was marked guarding and rigidity of the abdomen.

1. How should she be managed?
2. What is the differential diagnosis?
3. How should she have been managed before?

1. The most urgent requirement is resuscitation. An intravenous infusion should be commenced and at the same time blood taken for cross-matching with a minimum of four units requested. Shock of this degree in the absence of any external signs of bleeding implies an intra-abdominal haemorrhage of significant proportions and no time should be lost in transferring the patient to the operating theatre for laparotomy. Anaesthesia should be induced rapidly without waiting for the patient's vital signs to stabilise and the abdomen should be opened expeditiously. As soon as the site of bleeding has been found and clamped, the patient's general condition can be attended to and a central venous pressure line inserted. The subsequent surgical management will depend on the individual circumstance of the patient.

2. With clinical signs of shock as obvious as these, the most likely diagnosis is a ruptured ectopic pregnancy, but other acute haemorrhagic crises such as bleeding from a ruptured ovarian cyst or perforated ulcer are occasionally encountered. Sudden and rapid expulsion of an IUCD leading to cervical shock and acute septicaemia are possible but rare causes.

3. Any accident and emergency department doctor will testify to the frequency with which patients present with acute abdominal pain which settles spontaneously. When the patient has consumed an excess of alcohol this makes diagnosis more difficult as it is often impossible to obtain a satisfactory history, and many clinical signs may be masked or accentuated. Nevertheless there were sufficient factors in this particular case which should have suggested an ectopic pregnancy.

   The diagnosis should always be suspected in a young woman presenting with acute colicky pain. An IUCD in situ and a history of recent menstrual irregularity should increase this suspicion and the finding of tenderness on bimanual examination makes further investigation essential. Ultrasound scan has generally proved to be unsatisfactory for excluding ectopic pregnancy, but beta-hCG immunoassay will often be of value. The morbidity associated with ectopic pregnancy is such that, even when ultrasound and beta-hCG assay are available, admission to hospital for overnight observation is recommended.

Gynaecology 47

A 36-year-old telephonist, married with two children aged 19 and 17, was invited by her general practitioner to attend for a cervical smear. The practice records showed that she had never had one previously, but now that she was over 35 she fell within the Department of Health recommendations for cervical cytology. She had been on the oral contraceptive pill before her first pregnancy and for two years after the second one, when she finally persuaded her husband to have a vasectomy. She smoked about 25 cigarettes a day.

The cervical smear was reported as showing moderate dyskaryosis and she was therefore referred for colposcopy. This revealed a wide atypical transformation zone with areas of punctation and mosaicism which stained densely aceto-white. A biopsy was taken and subsequently reported as showing CIN II with evidence of wart virus infection. The lesion was treated by laser ablation to a depth of 7 mm.

At routine follow-up 6 months later the smear was still abnormal and repeat colposcopy this time suggested CIN III. This was confirmed histologically and the results discussed with the patient and her husband. Both were concerned that no guarantee could be given as to a cure and that frequent smears and possibly colposcopy would be required. They therefore requested that a hysterectomy be performed. This was carried out 3 weeks later and histologic examination of the cervix showed extensive CIN III in all blocks, but in two there was also evidence of stromal invasion to a depth of 5 mm. In addition, one area showed evidence of invasion into lymphatic vessels.

1. How often should routine cervical cytological screening be performed?
2. What risk factors for CIN existed in this case?
3. Having discovered invasive squamous carcinoma of the cervix after hysterectomy, what further measures would you suggest?

1. The Department of Health in the United Kingdom currently recommends (and will only pay for) cervical smears from women over 35 years of age and women over 30 with 3 or more children. Repeat smears should be performed at 5-year intervals. There is, however, much divergence of opinion as to the correct ages for, and frequency of, screening. The intercollegiate working party on cervical screening (RCOG, RC Path, RCGP and FCM), however, recommended screening at intervals of 3 years for all women between the ages of 20 and 64.

2. Risk factors in this case included two pregnancies before the age of 20, heavy cigarette smoking and prolonged use of the combined oral contraceptive pill. A further factor, missed until after the hysterectomy, was that both the woman and her husband had been treated for genital warts.

3. Had an invasive squamous carcinoma of the cervix been suspected before hysterectomy, a careful EUA and staging would have been required. If the tumour was no more than a stage I, a Wertheim hysterectomy could have been performed with a good chance of cure. Since this diagnosis had not been suspected before hysterectomy, the operation did not include pelvic lymphadenectomy or removal of a vaginal cuff. Computerised axial tomography showed no evidence of tumour spread and IVU was similarly normal, but it was felt that the theoretical risk of lymphatic involvement warranted external beam irradiation.

Gynaecology 48

A 39-year-old woman was referred to the gynaecological outpatient clinic by her general practitioner for investigation of worsening left iliac fossa pain and backache. Her symptoms had begun some months after a routine laparoscopic sterilisation, at which time no pelvic abnormality was noted and an occlusive (Falope) ring had been applied to each tube. The pain was initially associated with her periods, though subsequently it lasted throughout the menstrual cycle. The patient felt that her pain was becoming worse, was not relieved by anything she did, or by any medication she was given. The left iliac fossa pain had preceded the backache and was still the main cause for her concern. She was otherwise well with no urinary or bowel symptoms and she had continued to menstruate regularly.

On examination her general condition was good, there were no abdominal masses palpable, nor any tenderness elicited on deep palpation, and vaginal examination revealed normal pelvic organs with no masses or tenderness present. Urinalysis was clear and pelvic ultrasound scan confirmed the clinical findings. The woman was therefore reassured and discharged back to her general practitioner, no gynaecological abnormality having been detected.

Over the next three months the woman was referred to a general surgeon, a rheumatologist and a gastroenterologist, none of whom were able to find a cause for her pain which was now becoming much worse. She was finally referred to a urologist who elicited slight left loin pain and therefore arranged intravenous urography. This showed a left hydronephrosis and a dilated ureter extending down to the point where the ureter crossed under the left broad ligament. The urologist wrote to the gynaecologist who had performed the sterilisation advising him to contact his medical defence society.

1. What is the differential diagnosis in this case?
2. How would you manage it further?

1. The initial assumption on both the part of the patient and the urologist was that the ureteric blockage had been caused during the sterilisation procedure. It was suggested that, in picking up the fallopian tube on that side, the ureter might have been grasped inadvertently, or alternatively kinked by the application of the ring to the left tube. Other possibilities considered included retroperitoneal fibrosis, impacted fibroids or ovarian cysts, though these were not detected in this case. The presence of a stone in the ureter was discounted by the fixed position of the pain, the absence of any haematuria and the urographic findings.

2. The clinical situation calls for laparotomy and exploration of the lower ureteric course. This was duly performed jointly by the urologist and the gynaecologist with the hospital medical photographer in attendance. The first finding was that both tubes appeared to have been correctly occluded with minimal kinking of the broad ligaments. The uterus and ovaries were normal and there were no adhesions present in the pelvis. The left ureter was then exposed from the point at which it crossed the pelvic brim down towards the site of the obstruction. The left broad ligament was opened by dividing the left round ligament and the obstruction identified as a 2 cm diameter fixed and hard mass compressing the ureter and attached medially to the left cardinal ligament. It was removed with some difficulty and only after a hysterectomy and left salpingo-oophorectomy had been performed to give access. Left nephrectomy was also performed through a separate incision. The patient made an uneventful recovery.
The histology subsequently showed that the mass was an endometrioma.

A 29-year-old woman presented complaining of secondary infertility. She had 1 child, a boy, delivered by elective caesarean section 7 years earlier for a breech presentation. She had used a combined oral contraceptive pill for the subsequent 2 years when she began trying for a second pregnancy. After 2 years without success, she sought help and was duly referred for investigation.

There was no obvious cause for her infertility in her history and physical examination was normal. Her husband's semen analysis showed a count of 210 million with 60% motility at 2 hours and with 5% abnormal forms. Serum prolactin was 247 mu/l, day 23 plasma progesterone 15 nmol/l and thyroid function normal. A diagnostic laparotomy was performed and confirmed normal pelvic organs and patent fallopian tubes. No sepsis or endometriosis was seen. A working diagnosis of anovulation was made and she was started on clomiphene citrate 50 mg daily from the 2nd to the 6th days of her cycle inclusive. A temperature chart was commenced and over the first 3 treatment cycles the records were biphasic, but no pregnancy occurred. The patient continued on this regimen for another 4 months without success and then decided she would take a break from treatment.

She returned to the clinic 7 months later to say that she had only had 1 period since stopping the clomiphene and this had been 6 weeks later. Pregnancy tests on several occasions had been negative and ultrasound scan in the clinic showed a normal-sized uterus with no evidence of pregnancy and no visible ovarian follicles. Serum prolactin was 351 mu/l, plasma progesterone 12 nmol/l and serum FSH and LH greater than 40 u/l and 50 u/l respectively.

1. What is the most likely cause of her amenorrhoea?
2. What are her chances of conception?
3. What further treatment is necessary?

1. The most likely cause for her secondary amenorrhoea is ovarian failure or premature menopause. The diagnostic criterion is the raised serum FSH since the increased LH level could be associated with this, ovulation, or polycystic ovary syndrome (PCOS). Even without a raised serum FSH level, PCOS is unlikely because of the absence of any follicles on ultrasound scan.

2. Her chances of spontaneous conception must be regarded as almost non-existent although, rarely, ovulatory cycles do resume. A pregnancy is possible using a donated oocyte fertilised in vitro and inserted back into the uterus following treatment with oestrogen and progesterone to provide an endometrium capable of sustaining an embryo.

3. The necessity for further treatment is controversial. Without medical intervention this patient will undergo all the changes associated with the menopause. Because of her age, she is at an increased risk of osteoporosis and of the psychological and other physical effects of the climacteric compared with women who enter the menopause at the average age of 50 years. For this reason, most gynaecologists would agree that hormone replacement therapy is indicated. This woman needs only oestrogen to alleviate any symptoms and protect her from osteoporosis, but unopposed oestrogen therapy is contraindicated in a woman who still has her uterus because of the risk of endometrial hyperplasia and a progestogen should be given for 12 days every month to induce withdrawal bleeds.

Gynaecology 50

After suffering from recurrent cystitis for many years, a 63-year-old woman was referred to the gynaecology outpatient clinic for further investigation. The attacks occurred at least once a month and on each occasion culture of a mid-stream specimen of urine failed to grow any organism. She had therefore been treated empirically with a variety of antibiotics and encouraged to drink plenty of fluids, but this had little effect on the frequency of her attacks. There was no urinary incontinence and, provided she was not actually having an attack of cystitis, she had no nocturia. On closer questioning it transpired that the attacks of cystitis invariably followed coitus, which had lately become a fairly uncommon occurrence, much to the woman and her husband's mutual dissatisfaction.

General examination was normal and there were no abdominal masses present, nor was there any renal angle tenderness. Vaginal examination revealed a moderately atrophic genital tract. The vagina was somewhat narrowed with thin, smooth walls and no rugose pattern, but no prolapse was noted. The cervix was atrophic with petechial haemorrhages on its surface and the uterus and adnexa felt normal.

Full blood count was normal, as was a chest X-ray.

1. An intravenous urogram and cystoscopy were arranged. What could they be expected to show?
2. How would you treat her?

1. Repeated negative urine cultures and microscopy make an infective cause for this woman's symptoms unlikely and tuberculosis is unlikely because of the normal chest X-ray. Her symptoms are therefore more likely to be due to a combination of coitus and genital tract atrophy and so IVU and cystoscopy are unlikely to diagnose any abnormality other than atrophic change.

2. Treatment should be aimed at overcoming her oestrogen deficiency and this can be achieved by a variety of means. Since the basic problem is vaginal rather than systemic, local oestrogen therapy with intravaginal cream should be tried first. The patient should use the cream three or four times a week at night, using an applicator to instil the cream into the vagina, until the symptoms abate, and thereafter on a weekly or as-necessary basis. If the response to this is inadequate, then systemic oestrogens could be considered.

   This lady still has her uterus and is therefore theoretically at risk from unopposed oestrogen stimulation. Providing oestrogen cream is given vaginally no more than three to four times weekly vaginal bleeding is unlikely; if a higher dose is required, or it is felt that oral hormone replacement therapy is indicated, then a progestogen should be given for 12 days each month to induce withdrawal bleeds.

Index

Birthplans, 117
Birth weight and growth retardation, 22
Bladder neck descent, 260
Blood groups, 92
Blood pH estimation, fetal, 20
Blood transfusions, 132
  intrauterine, 92-93
  for sickle cell crisis, 177
Body mass index, 8, 104-105, 166
Breast feeding and HIV infection, 138
Breech presentation, 115-116,
British Institute of Radiology, 146
British Journal of Hospital Medicine, 4
British Journal of Obstetrics and Gynaecology, 3
British Medical Journal, 3
British National Library, 4
Broad-spectrum antibiotics, 180
  rheumatic heart disease, 69
Bromocriptine, 148
Bronte, Charlotte, 65
Brow presentation, 19-20
Buserelin, 170, 190

Caesarean section
  for dehiscence of scar, 112
  for herpes simplex infection, 52
  multiple pregnancy, 114
  placental insufficiency, 46
  scar, 22, 111-112
Candida albicans, 196
Carbimazole, 80
Carbon dioxide laser therapy, 182, 201
Carcinoembryonic antigen, 157
Carcinoma
  cervix, 11, 12-13, 118, 181-182, 255-256, 267-268, *see* also CIN
    prognosis, 205
    squamous cell, 201, 204, 256, 267-268
  endometrioid, 180
  endometrium, 241-242, 244
  in situ, 200
    vulva, 225
  squamous cell, 12, 201, 204, 256, 267-268
  vagina, 186
  vulva, 225, 228
Carcinoma antigen, 125, 218
Cardiac anomalies, 124
Cardiac failure, 67, 69
Cardiac output in pregnancy, 68
Cardiac surgery, 68
Cardiotocography, 123-124

antepartum haemorrhage, 122
Caruncle, urethral, 210
Case history, taking, 1-2
Central chest pain, 175-176
Cephalopelvic disproportion, 76, 104
  relative, 128
Cervical intra-epithelial neoplasia
  (CIN), 11, 12, 13, 118, 181-182, 200, 255-256, 267
Cervix
  biopsy, 118
  carcinoma *see* Carcinoma, cervix
  cytological screening, 267-268
  duplication, 108
  dyskaryosis, 117-118, 199-200, 255-256, 267
  examination in preterm labour, 26
  forcible dilatation, 35
  metaplasia, squamous cell, 199-200
  neoplasms, 255-256, *see* also
    Carcinoma, cervix; Cervical
    intra-epithelial neoplasia
  polyps, 207-208
  smears, 117-118, 255, 267
  sutures, 35-36
Chancroid, 186
Chest pain, central, 175-176
Chlamydia trachomatis, 186
Chlorambucil, 152
Chlorpromazine, 64
Choriocarcinoma, 218
Chorionic villus aspiration, 30
Chromosomal anomalies, 54
CIN *see* Cervical intra-epithelial
  neoplasia
Cisplatin, 154
Clear cell adenocarcinoma of vagina, 12
Clomiphene, 35, 167-168, 170
Cloquet's node, 228
Clue cells, 194
Coagulation, failure, 32, 141-142
Coagulopathy, 143-144
  consumptive, 34, *see* also Diffuse
    intravascular coagulopathy
Cold cautery, 200-201
Colposcopy, 117-118, 200-201, 255, 267
Combined oral contraceptive, 179, 196, 230, 268
Compression of head, 27
Computer searches, 4-5
Cone biopsy in pregnancy, 118, 256
Congenital anomalies *see* Anomalies, congenital
Congenital HIV infection, 138-139
Congestive cardiac failure, 67, 69

Radiotherapy *(contd)*
  squamous cell carcinoma of vulva,
    228
Rapid adsorbent monoclonal
    antibody pregnancy test,   264
Real time ultrasound examination of
    fetal heart,   84
Rectocoele,   214
Recurrent cystitis,   273
Recurrent failure of placentation,   46
Recurrent miscarriage,   35-37,
    237-239
Recurrent urinary tract infection,
    99-101
Red degeneration of fibroids,   60,
    134, 190
References, finding,   3
Research,   3
Research workers,   4
Resection of ovaries,   170
Resuscitation of mother,   44
Retained products of conception,
    evacuation,   126, 144
Retention of urine, acute,   173-174
Retro peritoneal fibrosis,   270
Reversal of sterilisation,   149-150
Rhesus isoimmunisation,   91-93
Rheumatic heart disease,   67-69
Ring pessaries,   214
Robert's sign,   84
Rotation of head for malpresentation,
    18, 128
Rupture of membranes, premature,
    114
Rupture of uterus,   22, 112

Salbutamol,   37
Salpingitis and IUCD,   194
Sarcomatous change in fibroids,
    191
Scar dehiscence,   111
Scar of caesarean section,   22,
    111-112
Schiller's iodine test,   182, 201
Scintigraphy,   80, 130
Screening, cervical,   267-268
Sebaceous cysts of vulva,   212
Secondary infertility,   249
Selective fetocide,   114
Septa
  uterus,   110
  vagina,   108
Sexual abuse,   258
Sexually transmitted disease,   194,
    221, *see also specific diseases*
Shock,   44, 172, 175-177, 265-266
Shoulder
  dystocia,   109-110

pain,   171-172
presentation,   45
Sickle cell disease,   29-30, 176-177
Skene's glands,   212
Small fetus,   7-9
Small for dates,   125
Smith O W & Smith G Van S,   12
Smoking,   51-52, 120, 230, 268
Soft sore,   186
Spalding's sign,   84
Special care baby units,   122
Spina bifida,   120
Squamo columnar junction,
    199-200, 255
Squamous cell carcinoma,   12
  cervix,   201, 204, 256, 267-268
  vulva,   228
Squamous cell metaplasia of cervix,
    199-200
Stafl A,   12
Staging
  carcinoma of cervix,   203-204
  squamous cell carcinoma of vulva,
    228
Stature of parents,   103-105
Stein-Leventhal syndrome,   170
Sterilisation,   149-150, 161-162, 172,
    269-270
  reversal,   113
  rheumatic heart disease,   69
Steroids, topical therapy,   224-225
Stilboestrol,   11-12
Stillbirth,   16
Strawberry vagina,   196
Stress incontinence, genuine,
    259-260
Subacute bacterial endocarditis,   68
Subglottic stenosis,   46
Submucous fibroids,   190
Subseptate uterus,   108
Suction cannula for termination of
    pregnancy,   179-180
Suction curettage,   234
Sulphamethoxazole,   101
Sulphur granules,   221
Superfetation,   54
Suprapubic discomfort and IUCD,
    194
Surgery, cardiac,   68
Sweat glands, apocrine, of vulva,
    212
Swollen leg in pregnancy,   129
Sympathomimetic drugs, beta-2,   37
Syntometrine,   132
Syphilis,   136, 186, 238

Tachycardia, fetal,   123-124
Tampons,   186-187

Vagina *(contd)*
  dysplasia, 181-182
  examination, 160
  foreign bodies, 258
  infantile, 257
  infection, 36
  neoplasms, 186
  pH, 258
  prepuberty, 257
  prolapse, 214-215
  septa, 108
  ulceration, 185-187
Vaginitis, 258
Valproic acid, 89
Vanillyl mandelic acid, 71-72
Varicose veins, progestogen-only oral
    contraceptive for, 150
VDRL (venereal disease research
    laboratory test), 135-136
Veganism, 22
Venereal disease in Pregnancy, 136
Venereal disease research laboratory
    test (VDRL), 135-136
Venography, 130
Venous thrombosis, 151-152
  deep, 130, 176
Ventilation, artificial, 46
Ventouse delivery, 128
Viral enteritis, 180
Visual field defects, 167-168
Vomiting in pregnancy, 63-65
Vulva
  biopsy, 224
  carcinoma, 228

  in situ, 225
  cysts, 211-212
  dystrophy, 224
  intraepithelial neoplasia, 225
  neoplasms, 227-228
Vulvitis
  acute, 51-52
  ulcerative, 25-26
Vulvovaginitis infantile, 258

Wart virus, 255-256
Wedge biopsy of cervix, 204
Wedge resection of ovaries, 170
Weight
  gain in pregnancy, 8, 58
  vs height, 8
  low, 166
  maternal, 104
Wertheim's hysterectomy, 205,
    268
White epithelium, 200
Withdrawal bleed, 179

Workers, research, 4

X-rays, *see also* Pelvimetry
  in early pregnancy, 145-146
  of fetus, 76
  for intrauterine death, 84
  in labour, 20
  for lost IUCD, 252

Yaws in pregnancy, 136